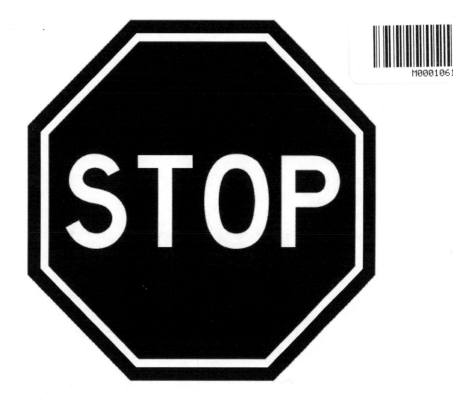

M000106193

FREE Test Taking Tips DVD Offer

To help us better serve you, we have developed a Test Taking Tips DVD that we would like to give you for <u>FREE</u>. **This DVD covers world-class test taking tips that you can use to be even more successful when you are taking your test.**

All that we ask is that you email us your feedback about your study guide. Please let us know what you thought about it – whether that is good, bad or indifferent.

To get your **FREE Test Taking Tips DVD**, email <u>freedvd@studyguideteam.com</u> with "FREE DVD" in the subject line and the following information in the body of the email:

    a.   The title of your study guide.

    b.   Your product rating on a scale of 1-5, with 5 being the highest rating.

    c.   Your feedback about the study guide. What did you think of it?

    d.   Your full name and shipping address to send your free DVD.

If you have any questions or concerns, please don't hesitate to contact us at <u>freedvd@studyguideteam.com</u>.

Thanks again!

MBLEx
Study Guide
2016

Table of Contents

Quick Overview

As you draw closer to taking your exam, preparing becomes more and more important. Thankfully, you have this study guide to help you get ready. Use this guide to help keep your studying on track and refer to it often.

This study guide contains several key sections that will help you be successful on your exam. The guide contains tips for what you should do the night before and the day of the test. Also included are test-taking tips. Knowing the right information is not always enough. Many well-prepared test takers struggle with exams. These tips will help equip you to accurately read, assess, and answer test questions.

A large part of the guide is devoted to showing you what content to expect on the exam and to helping you better understand that content. Near the end of this guide is a practice test so that you can see how well you have grasped the content. Then, answers explanations are provided so that you can understand why you missed certain questions.

Don't try to cram the night before you take your exam. This is not a wise strategy for a few reasons. First, your retention of the information will be low. Your time would be better used by reviewing information you already know rather than trying to learn lots of new information. Second, you will likely become stressed as you try to gain large amount of knowledge in a short amount of time. Third, you will be depriving yourself of sleep. So be sure to go to bed at a reasonable time the night before. Being well-rested helps you focus and remain calm.

Be sure to eat a substantial breakfast the morning of the exam. If you are taking the exam in the afternoon, be sure to have a good lunch as well. Being hungry is distracting and can make it difficult to focus. You have hopefully spent lots of time preparing for the exam. Don't let an empty stomach get in the way of success!

When travelling to the testing center, leave earlier than needed. That way, you have a buffer in case you experience any delays. This will help you remain calm and will keep you from missing your appointment time at the testing center.

Be sure to pace yourself during the exam. Don't try to rush through the exam. There is no need to risk performing poorly on the exam just so you can leave the testing center early. Allow yourself to use all of the allotted time if needed.

Remain positive while taking the exam even if you feel like you are performing poorly. Thinking about the content you should have mastered will not help you perform better on the exam.

Once the exam is complete, take some time to relax. Even if you feel that you need to take the exam again, you will be well served by some down time before you begin studying again. It's often easier to convince yourself to study if you know that it will come with a reward!

Test-Taking Strategies

1. Predicting the Answer

When you feel confident in your preparation for a multiple-choice test, try predicting the answer before reading the answer choices. This is especially useful on questions that test objective factual knowledge or that ask you to fill in a blank. By predicting the answer before reading the available choices, you eliminate the possibility that you will be distracted or led astray by an incorrect answer choice. You will feel much more confident in your selection if you read the question, predict the answer, and then find your prediction among the answer choices. After using this strategy, be sure to still read all of the answer choices carefully and completely. If you feel unprepared, you should not attempt to predict the answers. This would be a waste of time and an opportunity for your mind to wander in the wrong direction.

2. Reading the Whole Question

Too often, test takers scan a multiple-choice question, recognize a few familiar words, and immediately jump to the answer choices. Test authors are aware of this common impatience, and they will sometimes prey upon it. For instance, a test author might subtly turn the question into a negative, or he or she might redirect the focus of the question right at the end. The only way to avoid falling into these traps is to read the entirety of the question carefully before reading the answer choices.

3. Looking for Wrong Answers

Long and complicated multiple-choice questions can be intimidating. One way to simplify a difficult multiple-choice question is to eliminate all of the answer choices that are clearly wrong. In most sets of answers, there will be at least one selection that can be dismissed right away. If the test is administered on paper, the test taker could draw a line through it to indicate that it may be ignored; otherwise, the test taker will have to perform this operation mentally or on scratch paper. In either case, once the obviously incorrect answers have been eliminated, the remaining choices may be considered. Sometimes identifying the clearly wrong answers will give the test taker some information about the correct answer. For instance, if one of the remaining answer choices is a direct opposite of one of the eliminated answer choices, it may well be the correct answer. The opposite of obviously wrong is obviously right! Of course, this is not always the case. Some answers are obviously incorrect simply because they are irrelevant to the question being asked. Still, identifying and eliminating some incorrect answer choices is a good way to simplify a multiple-choice question.

4. Don't Overanalyze

Anxious test takers often overanalyze questions. When you are nervous, your brain will often run wild causing you to make associations and discover clues that don't actually exist. If you feel that this may be a problem for you, do whatever you can to slow down during the test. Try taking a deep breath or counting to ten. As you read and consider the question, restrict yourself to the particular words used by the author. Avoid thought tangents about what the author *really* meant, or what he or she was *trying* to say. The only things that matter on a multiple-choice test are the words that are actually in the question. You must avoid reading too much into a multiple-choice question, or supposing that the writer meant something other than what he or she wrote.

5. No Need for Panic

It is wise to learn as many strategies as possible before taking a multiple-choice test, but it is likely that you will come across a few questions for which you simply don't know the answer. In this situation, avoid panicking. Because most multiple-choice tests include dozens of questions, the relative value of a single wrong answer is small. Moreover, your failure on one question has no effect on your success elsewhere on the test. As much as possible, you should compartmentalize each question on a multiple-choice test. In other words, you should not allow your feelings about one question to affect your success on the others. When you find a question that you either don't understand or don't know how to answer, just take a deep breath and do your best. Read the entire question slowly and carefully. Try rephrasing the question a couple of different ways. Then, read all of the answer choices carefully. After eliminating obviously wrong answers, make a selection and move on to the next question.

6. Confusing Answer Choices

When working on a difficult multiple-choice question, there may be a tendency to focus on the answer choices that are the easiest to understand. Many people, whether consciously or not, gravitate to the answer choices that require the least concentration, knowledge, and memory. This is a mistake. When you come across an answer choice that is confusing, you need to give it extra attention. A question might be confusing because you do not know the subject matter to which it refers. If this is the case, don't eliminate the answer before you have affirmatively settled on another. When you come across an answer choice of this type, set it aside as you look at the remaining choices. If you can confidently assert that one of the other choices is correct, you can leave the confusing answer aside. Otherwise, you will need to take a moment to try to better understand the confusing answer choice. Rephrasing is one way to tease out the sense of a confusing answer choice.

7. Your First Instinct

Many people struggle with multiple-choice tests because they overthink the questions. If you have studied sufficiently for the test, you should be prepared to trust your first instinct once you have carefully and completely read the question and all of the answer choices. There is a great deal of research to suggest that the mind can come to the correct conclusion very quickly once it has obtained all of the relevant information. At times, it may seem to you as if your intuition is working faster even than your reasoning mind. This may in fact be true. The knowledge you obtain while studying may be retrieved from your subconscious before you have a chance to work out the associations that support it. Verify your instinct by working out the reasons that it should be trusted.

8. Key Words

Many test takers struggle with multiple-choice questions because they have poor reading comprehension skills. Quickly reading and understanding a multiple-choice question requires a mixture of skill and experience. To help with this, try jotting down a few key words and phrases on a piece of scrap paper. Doing this concentrates the process of reading and forces the mind to weigh the relative importance of the question's parts. In selecting words and phrases to write down, the test taker thinks about the question more deeply and carefully. This is especially true for multiple-choice questions that are preceded by a long prompt.

9. Subtle Negatives

One of the oldest tricks in the multiple-choice test writer's book is to subtly reverse the meaning of a question with a word like *not* or *except*. If you are not paying attention to each word in the question, you can easily be led astray by this trick. For instance, a common question format is, "Which of the following is…?" Obviously, if the question instead is, "Which of the following is not….?," then the answer will be quite different. Even worse, the test makers are aware of the potential for this mistake and will include one answer choice that would be correct if the question were not negated or reversed. A test taker who misses the reversal will find what he or she believes to be a correct answer and will be so confident that he or she will fail to reread the question and discover the original error. The only way to avoid this is to practice a wide variety of multiple-choice questions and to pay close attention to each and every word.

10. Reading Every Answer Choice

It may seem obvious, but you should always read every one of the answer choices! Too many test takers fall into the habit of scanning the question and assuming that they understand the question because they recognize a few key words. From there, they pick the first answer choice that answers the question they believe they have read. Test takers who read all of the answer choices might discover that one of the latter answer choices is actually *more* correct. Moreover, reading all of the answer choices can remind you of facts related to the question that can help you arrive at the correct answer. Sometimes, a misstatement or incorrect detail in one of the latter answer choices will trigger your memory of the subject and will enable you to find the right answer. Failing to read all of the answer choices is like not reading all of the items on a restaurant menu. You might miss out on the perfect choice.

11. Spot the Hedges

One of the keys to success on multiple-choice tests is paying close attention to every word. This is never more true than with words like *almost, most, some,* and *sometimes*. These words are called "hedges", because they indicate that a statement is not totally true or not true in every place and time. An absolute statement will contain no hedges, but in many subjects, like literature and history, the answers are not always straightforward. There are always exceptions to the rules in these subjects. For this reason, you should favor those multiple-choice questions that contain hedging language. The presence of qualifying words indicates that the author is taking special care with his or her words, which is certainly important when composing the right answer. After all, there are many ways to be wrong, but there is only one way to be right! For this reason, it is wise when taking a multiple-choice test to avoid answers that are absolute. An absolute answer is one that says things are either all one way or all another. They often include words like *every, always, best,* and *never*. If you are taking a multiple-choice test in a subject that doesn't lend itself to absolute answers, be on your guard if you see any of these words.

12. Long Answers

In many subject areas, the answers are not simple. As already mentioned, the right answer often requires hedges. Another common feature of the answers to a complex or subjective question are qualifying clauses, which are groups of words that subtly modify the meaning of the sentence. If the question or answer choice describes a rule to which there are exceptions or the subject matter is complicated, ambiguous, or confusing, the correct answer will require many words in order to be expressed clearly and accurately. In essence, you should not be deterred by answer choices that seem excessively long. Oftentimes, the author of the text will not be able to write the correct answer without offering some qualifications and modifications. As a test taker, your job is to read the answer choices thoroughly and completely and to select the one that most accurately and precisely answers the question.

13. Restating to Understand

Sometimes, a question on a multiple-choice test is difficult not because of what it asks but because of how it is written. If this is the case, restate the question or answer choice in different words. This process serves a couple of important purposes. First, it forces you to concentrate on the core of the question. In order to rephrase the question accurately, you have to understand it well. Rephrasing the question will concentrate your mind on the key words and ideas. Second, it will present the information to your mind in a fresh way. This process may trigger your memory of some useful scrap of information picked up while studying.

14. True Statements

Sometimes an answer choice will be true in itself, but it does not answer the question. This is one of the main reasons why it is essential to read the question carefully and completely before proceeding to the answer choices. Too often, test takers skip ahead to the answer choices and look for true statements. Having found one of these, they are content to select it without reference to the question above. Obviously, this provides an easy way for test makers to play tricks. The savvy test taker will always read the entire question before turning to the answer choices. Then, having settled on a correct answer choice, he or she will refer to the original question and ensure that the selected answer is relevant. The mistake of choosing a correct-but-irrelevant answer choice is especially common on questions related to specific pieces of objective knowledge, like historical or scientific facts. A prepared test taker will have a wealth of factual knowledge at his or her disposal, but may be careless in its application.

15. No Patterns

One of the more dangerous ideas that circulate about multiple-choice tests is that the correct answers tend to fall into patterns. These erroneous ideas range from a belief that B and C are the most common right answers, to the idea that an unprepared test-taker should answer "A-B-A-C-A-D-A-B-A." It cannot be emphasized enough that pattern-seeking of this type is exactly the WRONG way to approach a multiple-choice test. To begin with, it is highly unlikely that the test maker will plot the correct answers according to some predetermined pattern. The questions are scrambled and delivered in a random order. Furthermore, even if the test maker was following a pattern in the assignation of correct answers, there is no reason why the test maker would know which pattern he or she was using. Any attempt to discern a pattern in the answer choices is a waste of time and a distraction from the real work of taking the test. A test taker would be much better served by extra preparation before the test than by reliance on a pattern in the answers.

FREE DVD OFFER

Don't forget that doing well on your exam includes both understanding the test content and understanding how to use what you know to do well on the test. We offer a completely FREE Test Taking Tips DVD that covers world class test taking tips that you can use to be even more successful when you are taking your test.

All that we ask is that you email us your feedback about your study guide. To get your **FREE Test Taking Tips DVD**, email freedvd@studyguideteam.com with "FREE DVD" in the subject line and the following information in the body of the email:

    a. The title of your study guide.
    b. Your product rating on a scale of 1-5, with 5 being the highest rating.
    c. Your feedback about the study guide. What did you think of it?
    d. Your full name and shipping address to send your free DVD.

Anatomy and Physiology

Integumentary system

The primary structure of the integumentary system is the skin, which is composed of two layers: the epidermis and the dermis. The epidermis is the external layer of skin, and it is composed of five layers. From the inside out, they are the stratum germinativum, stratum spinosum, stratum granulosum, stratum lucidum, and stratum corneum. Skin cells are formed in the deepest layer and gradually move outward until they die and are removed from the body. The dermis contains the nerves, blood vessels, and sensory receptors. Nails, hair, and cutaneous glands are also part of the integumentary system. There are two kinds of cutaneous glands: sebaceous (oil-secreting) and sudoriferous (sweat-secreting). The integumentary system carries out numerous functions in addition to protecting the internal organs from injury and infection. The integumentary system contains nerves, which relay information about the external world to the brain. The skin contains sudoriferous and sebaceous glands that secrete sweat and oil, respectively. These chemicals help to regulate the amount of water in the body. The skin also adjusts its circulation and production of sweat in order to maintain a healthy body temperature. Finally, a small amount of oxygen is taken into the body through the skin, while a small amount of carbon dioxide is released from the skin.

Respiratory system

The respiratory system is designed to acquire necessary nutrients for the cells through respiration. Respiration is the process by which the body exchanges carbon dioxide wastes from the body for fresh oxygen. This gaseous exchange occurs in three separate areas:

- One area where the exchange occurs is deep inside the lungs, which is where the blood carries the carbon dioxide wastes to exchange them with the oxygen from the external environment.
- The internal respiration process is completed when the blood carries fresh oxygen to tissue cells throughout the body and then makes the transfer.
- Respiration also occurs within the individualized cells.

Respiration process

Respiration begins with the intake of oxygen through the nasal passages. It is then carried through the trachea, becoming moistened and filtered along the way. Once in the bronchi, it divides into the smaller bronchial trees, moving farther along until it reaches the alveoli, a tiny cluster of air sacs located at the end of the air passages. Tiny capillaries and arteries surround the alveoli. Through the process of diffusion, the carbon dioxide and oxygen are exchanged, thus allowing the oxygen to enter the bloodstream, where it is then carried throughout the body. The carbon dioxide is exhaled back into the environment.

Upper respiratory tract

The respiratory system is typically divided into the upper and lower respiratory tracts. The upper respiratory tract is composed of the nose, nasal cavity, pharynx, larynx, and upper trachea. The nose and nasal cavity warm the air as it enters the body. These components contain olfactory sensors for smelling. The pharynx is a tube through which air and food pass. The larynx, otherwise known as the voice box, sits behind the pharynx. It contains vocal cords, which vibrate and create sound when air passes through them. The trachea connects the larynx to the lungs. The trachea cleans air before it enters the lungs.

Lower respiratory tract

The lower respiratory tract consists of the lower trachea, bronchi, alveoli, and lungs. At the point that the trachea meets the lungs, it branches in two. It enters the lungs through the bronchi, which are treelike structures found inside the lungs. Bronchi are composed of smooth muscle, which expands and contracts during respiration. The smallest branches of the bronchi are called bronchioles. At the end of each bronchiole, there is an alveolus. Alveoli are tiny, clustered structures that introduce oxygen into the bloodstream and move carbon dioxide from the blood to the lungs for exhalation. The lungs are located on top of the diaphragm. They expand and contract during respiration.

Urinary system

The urinary system is composed of the kidneys, ureters, bladder, and urethra. The kidneys are located behind the stomach on either side of the backbone. The kidneys are susceptible to damage if a person experiences a blow or impact to the back. The ureters are foot-long tubes that carry urine from the kidneys into the urinary bladder, which is composed of three distinct layers of smooth muscle tissue. The bladder can expand to a maximum length of about five inches. Urine is expelled from the body through the urethra. The sphincter controls the dilations and contractions of the urethra.

Skeletal system

The skeletal system is composed of around 200 bones that, along with the attached ligaments and tendons, create a protective and supportive network for the body's muscles and soft tissues. There are two main components of the skeletal system: the axial skeleton and the appendicular skeleton. The axial skeleton includes the skull, spine, ribs, and sternum; the appendicular skeleton includes the pelvis and shoulders, and the various arm and leg bones attached to these. There are few differences between the male and female skeleton. The bones of the male tend to be a bit larger and heavier than those of the female, who will have a wider pelvic cavity (for childbirth). The skeleton does not move; it is pulled in various directions by the muscles.

The skeletal system consists of calcified structures under the skin that combine to form the framework for the human body. The skeletal system has five main functions. They are:
- To provide the framework for the body, provide support, and give the body its shape
- To serve as an additional form of protection for the internal organs, which are situated within the interior of this structure
- To provide a place for muscles to attach and to aid with movements of the body's limbs and appendages
- To assist in the production of red blood cells, which are formed in bone marrow
- To serve as a storage facility for minerals such as calcium phosphate, sodium, and magnesium

Digestive system

The digestive system is composed of organs that work to turn food into energy. This process begins with the teeth, which grind food into small particles. This makes food easier to digest. Food is then carried through the pharynx (throat) and esophagus to the stomach. In the stomach, it is partially digested by strong acids and enzymes. From there, food will pass through the small and large intestines, the rectum, and finally the anus. On this journey, it will mix with numerous chemicals so that it can be absorbed into the blood and lymph system. Some food will be converted into immediate energy, while some will be stored for future use. Whatever cannot be used by the body is expelled as waste.

Muscular system

The muscles of the body are attached to the skeleton by tendons and other tissues. Muscles exert force and move the bones of the body by contracting. Chemical energy is required for all muscular contractions. Every muscular act is the result of the shortening of one or more muscles. The muscles themselves are composed of millions of tiny proteins. Muscles are linked by nerves to the brain and spinal cord. There are three types of muscles. Cardiac muscles, which are found only in the heart, pump blood through the body. Smooth muscles can surround internal organs or be a component of them. Skeletal muscles are those which a person has voluntary control over. Skeletal muscles are the most common tissue in the body, accounting for between 25 and 40% of an individual's total body weight.

The muscular system is responsible for moving the skeleton. Muscles are considered organs within the muscular system. They are composed of cells and fibers that have the ability to stretch, lengthen, and constrict, depending on the needs of the human body. Muscles are responsible for the movement of the human body. The brain also plays a role in the body's movement by sending signals to the body. Muscles are the basis for all movements, including walking, flexing arms, grasping, breathing, and digesting food. They are also are responsible for the beating of the heart and the passage of the blood through the body. Muscles help to provide shape to the skeletal system and keep the body in an upright position. All of the muscles in the average human body account for approximately 40% to 60% of a person's total body weight. There are over 600 different muscles in the human body, and each carry out specific functions. Muscles utilize energy from food that is eaten and oxygen that is inhaled. The muscle is able to move and keep the body warm by using this energy. When muscles are overexerted and pushed beyond their limitations, massage can be beneficial because it can help the body release toxins.

Axial skeleton and appendicular skeleton

The axial skeleton is composed of the head and trunk areas of the human body. It is further broken down into the following regions: cranium, face, hyoid bone, ear, vertebral column, and the thoracic cage. The purpose of the axial skeleton is to protect the areas of the body that contain vital organs. There are approximately 80 separate bones contained within this skeletal system. The appendicular skeleton controls the movements of the upper and lower extremities. It is composed of the following structures: shoulder girdle, arm, hand, pelvic girdle, leg, and foot. There are a total of 126 separate bones located within this system. Although these bones move more freely than those of the axial skeleton, it is important for the massage therapist to consider any limitations in range of motion when performing a massage. In total, there are 206 bones in the human body,

Nervous system

The nervous system collects information for the body and indicates what the body should do to survive in the present conditions. For instance, it is the nervous system that sends a bad feeling when the body is cold, and then sends a more positive feeling when a person warms up. These important messages are sent by nerves, which vary in size and cover the entire body. The central nervous system is composed of the brain and spinal cord. The peripheral nervous system is composed of the rest of the body, including those organs which a person does not voluntarily control. The peripheral nervous system is divided into the sympathetic and parasympathetic systems, which counterbalance one another to allow for smooth functioning. The nervous system is composed of the various muscle groups. They are responsible for coordinating the body's activities, monitoring the organs of the body, and allowing the nerves to sense or perceive feeling and touch from all areas of the body. The main components of the nervous system include the brain, spinal cord, and nerves. The brain sends electrical impulses through the spinal cord to nerve endings throughout the body. These impulses control movement, sensations, feelings, and even thoughts. The nervous system controls the way that the body perceives input from internal and external sources. Nervous system movement can be either intentional or unintentional. The nervous system gives an organism the ability to process input received through the senses of sight, sound, taste, smell, and touch. It also allows the organism to carry out cognitive functions like moving, talking, and thinking.

Circulatory system

The circulatory system is composed of the heart, the blood vessels, and the blood. This system circulates blood throughout the body, provides nutrients and other essential materials to the body's cells, and removes waste products from the body. Arteries carry blood away from the heart, and veins carry blood back to the heart. Tiny capillaries found inside of the body's tissues distribute blood to the various cells in the body. The heart takes oxygenated blood from the lungs and circulates it throughout the body. When blood containing carbon dioxide returns to the heart, the carbon dioxide is sent to the lungs and expelled from the body. Other organs not always considered parts of the circulatory system (the kidneys and spleen for example) also help to remove some impurities from the blood.

The circulatory system is also known as the vascular system. The term "vascular" is defined as a vessel made up of a tube-like structure. These vessels help to transport fluids, such as blood or lymph, within the body of an organism. The circulatory system is responsible for an organism's circulation, a process which includes removing waste products and providing essential nutrients to tissues. The circulatory system can be divided into two separate systems. The first is the blood-vascular system, also known as the cardiovascular system. It consists of all the vessels used to transport blood, including veins, arteries, capillaries, and the heart. The second division is known as the lymph-vascular system, or lymphatic system. It includes the lymphoid organs, lymph nodes, lymph ducts, and the lymphatic vessels, which are used to transport lymph from the tissues to the circulatory system.

Blood
The average male human body is made up of about 11 pints of blood. Blood is a nutrient-filled fluid found in all areas of the body. It supplies nutrients to muscles, bones, ligaments, skin cells, etc. Blood is responsible for providing oxygen, water, and food to the body. Blood is also able to remove carbon dioxide and waste products from the body and send them through the excretory system to be eliminated from the body. Blood also helps to regulate the temperature of the body, allowing it to maintain an average temperature of 98.6 degrees Fahrenheit. When the body is injured, white blood cells within the vessels travel to the injured region to aid with healing. The red blood cells provide needed iron and help with coagulation in areas that are losing blood through hemorrhage. Blood is a type of connective tissue that is composed of 50-60% plasma.

Arteries, capillaries, and veins
The arteries, capillaries, and veins are tube-like structures that are responsible for the transportation of blood, lymph, and other substances throughout the body. The arteries are vessels that carry blood away from the heart. They help to carry fresh, oxygen-rich blood and other nutrients from the heart to other parts of the body. The veins carry blood, waste products, and carbon dioxide from the organs to the heart. Vein walls are thinner and less muscular than arteries. Veins also contain valves, which prevent the backwards flow of blood. Capillaries are blood vessels that are microscopic in size. They form a network that connects arterioles and venules. Because capillaries are only one cell layer thick, it is a simple process for wastes to pass readily into capillaries and for oxygenated, nutrient-rich blood to enter into organs.

Blood cells
Red blood cells deliver nutrients and oxygen to the body's tissues. Red blood cells are shaped like semi-flat, circular discs. They have the ability to alter their shape to maneuver through small channels. Certain diseases of the blood are caused by physiological changes to the red blood cells, and others are caused by an insufficient number of red blood cells within the body. Red blood cells are also known as erythrocytes. White blood cells are made within the bone marrow, and help the body's immune system fight off illnesses and injuries. An overproduction of white blood cells in the body can be an indication that certain diseases, such as leukemia, may be present. Therefore, an excessive number of white blood cells usually results in further medical testing. White blood cells help fight infection by encircling bacteria or producing antibodies. White blood cells are also known as leukocytes.

Diffusion and filtration
Capillaries form a network that connects arterioles and venules. They are thin-walled and have a high degree of permeability. Diffusion is the process in which a substance flows from an area that is higher in density to one that is lower. Capillaries carrying oxygen-rich blood filled with nutrients are denser than the tissues surrounding the capillary. The area within the tissues is filled with cellular waste and carbon dioxide. As the transfer occurs, the nutrients diffuse into the tissues, while the wastes diffuse into the capillaries. The wastes are then transported back to the heart. The wastes and carbon dioxide are released into the lungs for removal from the body. The blood is then filled with fresh, oxygenated blood. Filtration is the process in which the pressure of the blood forces the nutrients into the tissues and forces the wastes from the tissues into the capillaries. This is easily accomplished because of the thinness of the capillary walls.

Brain

The brain is composed of three segments: the cerebrum, the cerebellum, and the medulla oblongata, all of which interact with different parts of the nervous system. The cerebrum is located on the superior portion of the brain and is divided into the left and right hemispheres. The cerebrum is the largest section of the brain, and it is responsible for motor and sensory processes. The cerebrum is the area where higher learning thought processes take place. The cerebellum is located inferior to the cerebrum and just above the brain stem. The cerebellum is also responsible for motor and sensory actions, and can assist with maintaining balance and posture. The cerebellum influences an individual's attention span and their ability to process language and music. The cerebellum is also divided into two hemispheres. The medulla oblongata is the lowest part of the brain stem. It is located inferior to the cerebellum and superior to the spinal cord. The function of the medulla oblongata is to control the body's autonomic functions, including respiration, digestion, excretion, and cardiovascular functioning.

Bones

There are four types of bones that are part of the skeletal system. Long bones are those found in the arms, legs, and fingers. Short bones are those found in the carpals of the hand and tarsals of the foot. Flat bones are the pelvic bones, skull bones, and ribs. The irregular bones are commonly known as the vertebrae, and they are located in the spinal area. Although bone is considered a hard substance of the body, it is constantly evolving through regeneration. Bone is made up of about 33% animal (organic) matter and about 67 % mineral (earthy) matter. The organic matter includes bone cells, blood vessels, connective tissue, and bone marrow. Minerals found in bones include calcium phosphate and calcium carbonate. A long bone is composed of numerous layers. Each end is larger than the middle section, which allows this type of bone to move in conjunction with the bone nearest to it. The end of the bone is referred to as the epiphysis and is covered with a layer of cartilage called the articular cartilage. The purpose of this cartilage is to provide shock absorption. The long portion of the bone between the epiphysis is known as the diaphysis. The overall covering of the bone that is visible is called the periosteum. It is a network of fibers that protects the bone and is the area to which tendons and ligaments are attached. The next layer is made up of compact bone tissue, which forms the hard portion of the bone. The inner layer is called spongy bone. Bone marrow is located within this area, and it is also here that red blood cells are produced. The inner layer is known as spongy bone because it consists of empty spaces separated by thin, bony plates. The medullary cavity contains yellow bone marrow.

Reproductive system

The reproductive system consists of those organs and hormones that deal specifically with reproduction of the same type of organism. In humans and multi-celled organisms, this process is achieved sexually, which means both male and female organisms are required for successful reproduction to occur. In single-celled organisms, the process is called non-sexual or asexual reproduction, which means a partner is not required for reproduction to occur. In the human male, the purposes of the reproductive organs are to produce sperm, release male hormones, and perform the act necessary for reproduction. The male sexual organs include the penis, testes, vas deferens, prostate glands, seminal vesicles, and the bulbourethral glands. In the human female, the purpose of the reproductive organs is to provide for the development of the growing fetus after being impregnated by the male sperm. The organs of the female reproductive system include the ovaries, fallopian tubes, uterus, vagina, and the external genitalia.

Female reproductive system

Obviously, the main purpose of the female reproductive organs is to produce children. Each component of the reproductive system plays a part in this process. For instance, the reproductive system secretes the hormones estrogen and progesterone, which encourage the process of egg creation and fertilization. The reproductive organs also protect the developing fetus during its early development. The developing fetus is housed in the uterus. Once the fetus has developed sufficiently, a set of smooth muscles within the uterus dilate in order to allow the fetus to be delivered. The mammary glands, which produce milk for breast feeding, are also considered a part of the female reproductive system.

<u>Male reproductive system</u>
The primary function of the male reproductive system is to fertilize a female egg. Most of the structures within the male reproductive system, therefore, are either designed to produce sperm or to deliver sperm to a female. The male reproductive system produces testosterone, a hormone that stimulates sexual maturation during puberty. Testosterone is secreted by the testes, which also create sperm cells. Sperm cells leave the testes and enter the epididymis, where they develop until they are ejaculated. A set of smooth muscles in the tubes leading from the epididymis to the urethra propel sperm out of the urethra during ejaculation.

Special senses

The special senses are vision, hearing, smell, and taste (touch is described as a somatic sense). The visual system consists of the eyes and a series of nerves connecting the eyes to the brain. The external surface of the eye is composed of the lens, which is surrounded by the iris and covered by the cornea. The hearing system consists of the ear and the central auditory system. The system of smell, commonly known as the olfactory sense, is composed of various olfactory receptors in the nose, which transmit information about odors to the brain. The primary structure of the taste system is the tongue, which contains sensory receptors for the following kinds of tastes: sour, sweet, salty, savory, and bitter.

The functions of the various special senses should be fairly obvious. These senses are used to acquire information about the internal and external world of the person. The sense of sight is probably the most important of the special senses for human beings. It functions by allowing light to pass through the lens and hit the retina, after which the image is transmitted along the optic nerve to the brain. The sense of hearing basically functions as follows: sound waves are received through the ear. They vibrate the eardrum and then pass through a series of tubes, from which information is then transmitted to the brain through various auditory nerves. The system of taste depends on chemical reactions between receptors in the mouth and other materials, such as food and drink.

Heart

The heart is part of the cardiovascular system, which also consists of the blood vessels, capillaries, veins, and the blood itself. The heart is a four-chambered muscle, and its sole function is to pump oxygen-rich blood throughout the body. The heart is composed of the left atrium, right atrium, left ventricle, and right ventricle. The atria are the chambers located superior to the ventricles. The pathway through the heart is cyclical, meaning that the path through which the blood travels is a closed system. The veins carry the blood from the rest of the body to the heart, and it enters the heart through the right atrium. From there, it flows into the right ventricle. After it leaves the right ventricle, it travels past the pulmonary valve, entering the lungs. Here, the blood disposes of the body's wastes and gathers a fresh supply of oxygen from the lungs. It then reenters the heart through the left atrium. From here, the blood travels to the left ventricle, where the aorta helps to propel the oxygen-rich blood to the rest of the body.

Lymphatic system

The lymphatic system is connected to the cardiovascular system through a network of capillaries. The lymphatic system filters out disease-causing organisms, controls the production of disease-fighting antibodies, and produces white blood cells. The lymphatic system also prevents body tissues from swelling by draining fluids from them. Two of the most important components of this system are the right lymphatic duct and the thoracic duct. The right lymphatic duct circulates immunity-bolstering lymph fluid throughout the top half of the body, while the thoracic duct circulates lymph throughout the bottom half. The spleen, thymus, and lymph nodes all generate and store the chemicals found in lymph, which plays an essential role in protecting the body from disease.

The lymphatic system is also known as the lymph-vascular system. Lymph is a liquid made up primarily of white blood cells. Its makeup is similar to the interstitial fluid of the surrounding tissues, and it helps with the exchange of waste materials and nutrients from the tissues to the cells. Approximately 90% of the fluid is able to pass through the capillary walls and reenter the blood stream to return to the heart, but the last 10% contains particles that are too large to pass through these walls. Lymph fluid then collects these particles and transports them to the lymphatic ducts, where they are ultimately returned to the blood. Lymphatic massage has many benefits for the body, including helping the lymph nodes expel waste and increasing circulation. It also helps to clean tissues and aids in the production of lymphocytes, which improve the body's immune system response.

Lymph nodes
There are approximately 500-600 lymph nodes located in all areas of the body. They range in size, with the largest being about an inch long. Specifically, they can be found in the following regions:
- Back of the head – Assists with drainage of wastes from the scalp area
- Back and sides of the neck – Assists with drainage of mouth and nasal cavities
- Under the jaw – Helps to drain the mouth
- Along the upper extremities – Located under the armpit, in the crook of the elbow, and under the chest muscle
- Abdominal region – Located along the blood vessels in this area
- Lower extremities – Located in the groin and at the back of the knee

Immune system

The immune system is responsible for protecting the body from outside influences such as bacteria, toxins, and viruses. It also controls the response to any internal changes that occur in the body, such as the development of cancerous cells and tumors, as well as any illnesses caused by damage to the organs or tissues. The immune system responds by creating an antibody that works against the antigen, or "antibody-generating" substance, to render it inactive. Once an antigen is discovered in the body, the immune system creates antibody proteins that bind to the antigen and diminish its control over the body. There are two types of immunity. Innate immunity is present at birth. The degree to which this immunity is present depends on the amount of immunity inherited from the mother. The second type of immunity is acquired immunity. This type of immunity usually refers to immunity that is acquired as a result of a vaccination. Immunity acquired in this fashion can last for days, weeks, or even years, depending on the bacteria or virus being vaccinated against.

Endocrine system

The endocrine system creates and secretes hormones, which accomplish a wide variety of tasks in the body. The endocrine system is made up of glands. These glands produce chemicals that regulate metabolism, growth, and sexual development. Glands release hormones directly into the bloodstream, where they are then transported to the various organs and tissues of the body. It is generally accepted that the endocrine system is composed of the pituitary, thyroid, parathyroid, and adrenal glands, as well as the pancreas, ovaries, and testes. The endocrine system regulates its level of hormone production by monitoring the activity of hormones. When it senses that a certain hormone is active, it reduces or stops production of that hormone.

<u>Glands</u>
The endocrine system helps the nervous system to function properly by producing hormones to stimulate and regulate various processes of the body. The precise functions of the major glands in the endocrine system are as follows:

- Pituitary: This gland secretes hormones that encourage muscle and bone growth (growth hormone), releases adrenaline, initiates breast milk production, produces sex sells, and regulates the thyroid.
- Adrenal: The adrenal gland secretes epinephrine (adrenaline), norepinephrine, glucocorticoids, and mineralocorticoids. These hormones help the body deal with stress and conserve water, in addition to numerous other functions.
- Thyroid: This gland secretes hormones that control metabolism and regulate the amount of calcium in the blood.
- Parathyroid: The parathyroid gland helps regulate blood calcium levels.
- Thymus: The thymus aids in the production of immune cells.
- Pineal: This gland produces melatonin, which regulates the sleep/wake cycle.

<u>Hormones</u>
Hormones are chemical substances produced by the endocrine glands that have an influence on tissues or organs within the body. Hormones can lead to an increase in growth, can activate the immune system process, and can bring about the onset of changes such as puberty or menopause. Hormones are also responsible for initiating the fight or flight response to fear or other stimuli, such as stress. The body's metabolism is also regulated by hormonal changes. In addition, the release of hormones can help a woman's body maintain and carry a fetus to term and can also help with aftercare. The production of hormones can be caused by the release of other hormones, by environmental factors, or by activities occurring in the brain. Hormones play a key role in metabolic processes that enable the body to function.

Digestive system

The purpose of the digestive system is to digest food and also to absorb it so that it may be used by the body's tissues and organs for energy. The digestive system is made up of the alimentary canal and the accessory digestive organs. The alimentary canal is the gastrointestinal tract. It is made up of the following organs and body parts: mouth, pharynx, esophagus, stomach, small intestine, and large intestine. The accessory digestive organs are those that greatly assist with the digestive process, but play a secondary role. For example, the teeth, tongue, salivary glands, liver, pancreas, and gallbladder all aid in digestion, but the body can still process food without them. The process of digestion begins in the mouth, where the teeth aid in breaking down food particles into manageable pieces. After mastication, saliva helps to propel food down the esophagus and into the stomach. Here, acids break down the food further; the food then leaves the stomach to enter the small intestine. At this point, the food is broken down further and absorbed by the villi, small projections that line the small intestine. After this point, waste products are moved into the large intestine, where they are prepared for expulsion from the body through the rectum.

Excretory system

The excretory system is the system responsible for removing wastes from the body. This system does not just handle wastes that are produced by food absorption; it is also involved with removing respiratory wastes, such as carbon dioxide, and wastes excreted during the process of sweating. The organs that are considered part of the excretory system are the kidneys, sweat glands, lungs, and rectum. If these wastes are not excreted and remain in the body, they can cause serious health problems. The urinary system is composed of the kidneys, bladder, ureter, hilum, and urethra. As the body absorbs nutrients, wastes are sent to the kidneys for processing. From here, they travel to the bladder, where they are released from the body through the urethra. Noticeable changes in the color of the urine or in the measured amount released from the body can indicate damage elsewhere in the body. Urine can be tested for the presence of drugs, white blood cells, blood, glucose, and hormonal imbalances, and is therefore a good indicator of the body's overall health.

Healthcare Related and Medical Terminology

Root words

The following are the most common root words used in medical terminology: abdomin- (abdomen); angio- (vessel); arterio- (artery); arthr- (joint); brachi- (arm); cardi- (heart); cephal- (head); cerebr- (cerebrum); cervic- (neck); crani- (skull); dent- (teeth); dermat- (skin); fibr- (fiber); gastr- (stomach); gynec- (woman); hemat- (blood); hepat- (liver); hist- (tissue); myo- (muscle); neph- (kidney); neur- (nerve); oss-, osteo- (bone); ped- (child); pneumat- (breathing); pod- (foot); pulm- (lung); rhin- (nose); stern- (chest); thorac- (chest); ven- (vein); and vertebr- (spine). These words may or may not be preceded by a common medical prefix; they will almost certainly be followed by a common medical suffix.

Prefixes

The following are the most common prefixes used in medical terminology: ab- (away from); a-, an- (without); ad- (toward); ante- (before); anti- (against); bi- (two); circum- (around); contra- (against); de- (down, down from); dia- (across, through); dys- (difficult); epi- (over, upon); ex- (out of); extra- (beyond); hemi- (half); hetero- (other); homeo- (same); hyper- (above, high); hypo- (under, low); infra- (below); inter- (between); intra- (within); mal- (bad); mono- (one); poly- (many); post- (after); pre- (before, in front of); quad- (four); retro- (backward); sub- (under); super- (above, in addition to); supra- (over, above); syn- (together); trans- (across); and tri- (three).

Suffixes

The following are the most common suffixes used in medical terminology: -al (pertaining to a particular area); -algia (pain); -ar (pertaining to a particular area); -ase (enzyme); -cyte (cell); -ectomy (removal of); -emia (blood condition); -genic (producing); -gram (record of); -itis (inflammation of); -logy (study of); -oid (similar to); -oma (tumor); -osis (condition of); -pathy (disease); -phobia (irrational fear of); -plasty (surgical repair of); -plegia (paralysis); -scope (instrument for examining visually); -stomy (opening); and -tomy (incision). These suffixes are typically appended to the end of one of the common medical roots.

Metabolism, anabolism, and catabolism

Metabolism is the cellular process by which the cells take in nutrients, expel wastes, and perform their intended activities or functions. Virtually all chemical processes performed by the cell are metabolic. The breakdown of proteins, carbohydrates, and fats is part of the metabolic process.

Anabolism is one of the phases of metabolism. In an anabolic state, energy is used by the cells to build up amino acids and other substances into more complex organic compounds, such as enzymes.

During the next stage, catabolism, the larger molecules are broken down into smaller components to produce energy. One byproduct of this process is ATP (adenosine triphosphate), which stores energy until it is ready to be released.

Planes

Sagittal plane
In attempting to identify the sides of the body, it is important to understand the terminology that best describes the positioning of the body with relation to planes. There are three main planes to consider: sagittal, coronal, and transverse. These planes are commonly described using the following terminology: superior or inferior; anterior or posterior; and medial, lateral, distal, and proximal. When the body is positioned in such a way that the face is forward and the palms are facing up, an imaginary line is drawn vertically down the body, dividing it into left and right halves. This is referred to as the sagittal plane.

<u>Coronal plane</u>
When the body is divided into front and back halves, it is referred to as coronal. When the body is divided into upper and lower halves, it is referred to as transverse. Cranial is a synonym for superior, while caudal is a synonym for inferior. Anterior is a synonym for ventral, and posterior is a synonym for dorsal. Medial refers to any area pertaining to the midline of the body. Lateral refers to the part of the body farthest from the midline or center. Distal is the term used when speaking of the parts of the body farthest from a point of attachment. Proximal refers to the parts of the body nearest to the point of attachment.

Body cavities and organs

The ease with which one can recall the locations of body organs is dependent upon the individual's knowledge of the body's planes. The main body cavities are as follows: cranial, spinal, thoracic, abdominal, and pelvic.
- The cranial cavity encompasses everything relating to the skull.
- The spinal cavity is the portion of the body relating to the spinal column and the vertebrae.
- The thoracic cavity is divided into two sections. They relate to the heart and lungs, respectively.
- The abdominal cavity, the portion of the body located below the diaphragm, holds the liver, stomach, pancreas, spleen, and the intestines.
- Finally, the pelvic cavity houses parts of the reproductive system, the bladder, and the rectum.

Dorsal cavities are the cranial and spinal cavities. Ventral cavities are the thoracic, abdominal, and pelvic cavities.

Anterior regions of the body

- Frontal – refers to the head
- Temporal – refers to the temple of the skull, or, more precisely, to the temporal bone
- Cervical – refers to the neck
- Deltoid – refers to the shoulder area
- Axillary – refers to the armpit area, where the axillary gland is located
- Brachial – refers to the area between the elbow and shoulder
- Hypochondrium – refers to the abdominal area lateral from the epigastric (upper central abdominal) region
- Umbilical – refers to the area between the navel and pubic region
- Hypogastric – refers to the area under the stomach and above the umbilical region
- Patellar – refers to the knees and kneecap
- Femoral – refers to the femur or thigh
- Inguinal – refers to the groin
- Epigastric – refers to the abdominal region
- Pectoral – refers to the chest area

Posterior regions of the body

- Occipital – refers to the back of the head, an area which includes the occipital bone
- Parietal – refers to the head, posterior to the frontal and anterior to the occipital
- Mastoid – refers to the area behind the ear; the set of bones in this area is known as the mastoid process
- Cervical – refers to the neck
- Scapular – refers to the back of the shoulder or shoulder blade (known as the scapula)
- Lumbar – refers to the lower back
- Sacral – refers to the area below the lumbar region and between the gluteal, and specifically to the sacrum (tailbone)
- Gluteal – refers to the buttock muscles (known as the gluteus maximus and minimus)
- Popliteal – refers to the area behind the knee, including the hamstring

Anatomical parts of the body

The human body is divided into several distinct regions, which are the head, spine, trunk, and extremities.
- The head region encompasses the skull, face, eyes, nose, mouth, and chin.
- The spinal region is made up of the bones that support the head and trunk of the body, which include the vertebrae.
- The trunk region is divided into additional subcategories. One is the thoracic region, or chest. It contains the rib cage, heart, lungs, esophagus, and parts of the trachea. The second subcategory is the abdominal area, which contains the stomach, kidneys, liver, intestines, and diaphragm.
- The final region of the body is the extremities. These are the upper limbs, which are the shoulders, arms, wrists, and hands, as well as the lower limbs, which are the hips, thighs, legs, knees, ankles, and feet.

Groups of tissue

Tissues, which are composed of groups of cells that carry out similar functions, are found in every organ in the body. There are five main groups of tissues, and each carries out different functions.
- Epithelial – This type of tissue serves a protective function and can be further divided according to shape and the number of cell layers.
- Connective – This type of tissue is the framework for binding structures together.
- Muscular – This type of tissue is responsible for pulling together, or contracting, elongated cells, which causes body parts to move.
- Nervous – This type of tissue is composed of nerve cells, which are primarily located in the brain, spinal cord, and other nerves. It acts as a channel through which messages are sent to and from the brain.
- Liquid – This type of tissue includes blood and lymph. It circulates throughout the body, where it removes wastes and absorbs nutrients.

Epithelial tissue
The primary purpose of epithelial tissue is to form a protective layer or barrier against infections. This tissue also assists in the processes of absorption, waste excretion, and fluid secretion. It also helps protect the body against bacteria and injury. This type of tissue is found on all surfaces of the body, over the organs, and within the interior lining of the organs. Depending on the location, this tissue can be further subdivided into different categories of cells.
- Squamous cells are flat cells that are generally one cell thick.
- Cuboidal cells are square-shaped cells that can be many layers thick.
- Columnar cells are tall and rectangular.
- Stratified squamous cells are several layers thick and transitional squamous cells are generally flatter and closely packed together.

Connective tissue
Connective tissue binds the various parts of the body together. These tissues also help to provide the structural framework of the body. Connective tissue called areolar tissue connects the skin to other tissues and helps to fill the spaces within muscles. This tissue is found beneath the dermis, is present within the digestive tract, and can also be found under all epithelial tissue. This tissue is also referred to as superficial fascia. It contains numerous blood cells and nerves. Another type of connective tissue is adipose tissue, which is composed primarily of fat cells called adipocytes. Its function is to protect against heat loss and to store energy for the body. Primarily found in the largest quantities in the abdominal region, it can also exist near the heart muscle, around the kidneys, and virtually anywhere underneath the skin. Excess adipose tissue around the centralized region of a person's body increases their risk of developing certain health problems, including cardiovascular disease and diabetes mellitus.

Fascia: Fascia is the connective tissue that surrounds all portions of the body, including the skin, muscles, bones and joints. It serves a protective purpose, and also provides lubrication, shape, and support. Fascia is a fibrous network made of elastin and collagen that is embedded within a gel substance. It helps the body move and reduces the possibility of irritation. The fascia layer just beneath the skin is known as the superficial fascia. Deep fascia is located around each muscle tissue and fiber. It allows the muscles to move independently and also contract together as a unit. Deep fascia also helps muscles attach to bone. Subserous fascia is located between deep fascia and the membranes that line the internal cavities of the body. It helps to fill in some of the gaps, while still allowing for slight movement of the internal organs.

Tissue damage, injury, or infection

The body has a number of ways to fight tissue damage, injury, and infection. The cells release proteins such as histamines and cytokines to begin the healing process. This release coincides with the constriction of blood vessels, which helps to prevent excessive bleeding. Following this, capillaries dilate to allow for the influx of white blood cells and antibodies, which fill the injured area. Platelets and fibrin aid in stopping any bleeding and in preventing any potentially harmful matter from entering the blood. They begin the clotting process, which stops the bleeding. Any pathogens are inactivated by neutrophils and macrophages. Finally, collagen enters the area to repair and mend any damaged tissues by creating scar tissue. At this point, any inflammation will have begun to subside, and this usually happens within 72 hours. Scar tissue may continue to be produced for weeks or months, depending upon the severity of the injury. When there is inflammation, massage is not recommended because it impedes the healing process. After the swelling has subsided, however, massage helps to stimulate the production of scar tissue.

Tissue repair and healing
Surface tissue and skin generally require the least amount of recuperative time to heal and return to their original state. Deeper tissues, such as those within muscles, take longer to heal and require more in-depth stretching, friction, and massage techniques performed on those areas. Bones and ligaments tend to heal slowly, while muscles and tendons heal with considerable scarring and some loss of elasticity and strength. Portions of the central nervous system that have been injured or traumatized often do not heal at all. Correct techniques for the type of injury have been shown to alleviate pain and strengthen the muscles, ligaments, and tendons, thereby decreasing the amount of scar tissue formed. The development of scar tissue is caused by connective tissue cells that have entered the area of injury and developed a fiber network. This allows regenerative tissue to bond, which creates scar tissue. It is important to minimize the amount of scar tissue in any given area in order to prevent excessive buildup that can inhibit movement and range of motion.

Membranes

A membrane is the outermost layer of a cell. Membranes serve as barriers between the interiors and exteriors of cells. Membranes are divided into two main categories: epithelial membranes and fibrous connective tissue membranes. Epithelial membranes have an outer covering of epithelium, while fibrous connective tissue membranes are composed of binding fibers and a thick gel substance. There are two types of epithelial membranes: mucous and serous membranes. Mucous membranes produce a thick substance that helps protect and lubricate the cells and tissues. Serous membranes produce a liquid that also provides lubrication. The main serous membranes in the body are the pleura, pericardium, and peritoneum. Other membranes within the body are the skeletal membrane, the perichondrium, and the synovial membrane.

Ligaments

Ligaments are dense bundles of parallel fibers that connect one bone to another; this connection is commonly known as a joint. Ligaments are a part of the joint capsule. However, they may also attach to other nearby bones that are not a part of the joint. Ligaments differ from muscles in that they cannot contract. Instead, ligaments passively strengthen and support the joints by absorbing some of the tension that results from movement. Ligaments do contain nerve cells that are sensitive to the position and speed of movement of the ligament, and so it is possible for ligaments to hurt. One function of this pain is to alert the person if there is an unnatural or dangerous movement of the joint. Ligaments may also be strained or rupture if they are placed under unnecessary or violent stress.

Kinesiology

Muscle tissue

The purpose of muscle tissue is to contract the fibers that compose the muscles, which allows the body to move. The first type of muscle tissue is skeletal muscle. Tendons attach these muscles to the bones. Movement of these muscles is controlled through conscious effort. Impulses are sent from the brain and travel through the nerves to the muscle. Because of the manner in which impulses are transmitted, these skeletal muscles are referred to as voluntary muscles. The cells of these muscles are long and resemble threads. They contain dark and light markings known as striations. These types of muscles are known as striated muscles. A second type of muscle tissue is smooth muscle. Generally, this type is non-striated and cannot be controlled or made to contract through voluntary means. Food is transported through the digestive tract with the aid of smooth muscles. A third type of muscle tissue is cardiac muscle tissue, which is found only in the heart. It functions involuntarily, and helps to pump blood throughout the body via the arteries and veins through cardiac contractions.

Composition of skeletal muscle tissue
Skeletal muscle tissue is composed of fibrous tissue arranged in bundles called fascicles. These fascicles are made up of muscle fibers connected to one another through connective tissue. An extensive supply of blood and lymph vessels, capillaries, and nerve fibers are contained within skeletal muscle tissue. The muscle receives its supply of oxygen through the blood vessels. There are two types of skeletal muscle fibers: type I and type II. Type I muscle fibers are characterized by a large number of reddish fibers, which provide excellent endurance for the muscle through oxidative metabolism. Type II fibers are white in color, and are more suitable for shorter bursts of energy or when speed is required. They rely on anaerobic metabolism for energy and tire more easily. The composition of an individual's skeletal muscle tissue is determined by genetics and by the type of exercise they do on a regular basis.

Structure of muscle tissue
Muscle tissue is made up of bundles of fibers that are held in position and separated by various partitions. These partitions range from large (deep fascia, epimysium) to small (perimysium, endomysium), and often extend beyond the entire length of the muscle and form tendon, which is connected to another bone. Each muscle cell is extremely long, and has a large number of nuclei. Every muscle cell contains a number of smaller units called sarcomeres; these contain thick filaments of the protein myosin and thin filaments of the protein actin. Muscle tissue contracts when a nerve stimulates the muscle and the thin filaments compress within the sarcomere, causing a general muscle contraction.

Muscle shapes

The muscles of the human body can be numerous shapes, depending on their function. In the trapezius, for instance, the muscle fibers are arranged in a broad, flat pattern, and attach at a large number of points along the scapula. The bicep, on the other hand, is a long, narrow muscle. The muscles of the deep back are very short and appear as knotty bundles along the spinal column. Longer muscles are generally capable of producing highly visible external movements and are used to transport heavy objects, for example. Small, deep muscles are usually responsible for precise, balancing adjustments. Muscles that only cross over one joint are called monoarticular, while those that extend across and move more than one joint are called polyarticular.

Isometric and isotonic contractions

When reviewing the ways that muscles contract and expand, it is important to note the differences between the two types of muscle contractions. An isometric contraction occurs when the muscle is contracting, but no increase in the length of the muscle is observed. The muscle being isolated is tensed, but the corresponding body part does not move. An isotonic contraction occurs when the muscle contracts and the distance from one end of the muscle to the other changes. The majority of the body's voluntary movements are considered isotonic. Isometric contractions are responsible for keeping the body in an upright position. An isometric contraction occurs when a person pushes extremely hard against a heavy object, but is not able to move it. The tension felt within the body is considered an isometric contraction. When a person is engaged in regular physical exercise, such as running, the muscle contractions that occur are isotonic.

Muscle attachments

In most cases, a muscle is attached to two different bones. When the body moves, the origin bone will be fixed in some way, while the other bone (known as the insertion bone) moves because of a muscle contraction. Occasionally, health professionals will refer to the origin bone as the proximal bone. Although the only voluntary motion a muscle is capable of is contraction, muscles are generally elastic in nature, meaning that muscles stretched beyond their normal length will usually return to their original size. This is part of the reason why the body has a general tendency to retain a particular shape. Muscles can be attached to bones by tendons or muscle fibers.

Functions of muscles

Muscles are able to perform their various functions because they possess certain characteristics. These characteristics are described using the following terms: irritability, contractility, elasticity and extensibility. Irritability refers to the ability of muscles to receive and react to stimuli from outside the body, such as the touch of massage, or to respond to internal stimuli, such as electrical currents sent from the brain. The muscle's irritability also refers to their reaction to heat, chemicals such as acids or salts, and other impulses. Contractility refers to muscles that are capable of shortening and therefore exerting force. An example of a muscle that possesses contractility is the cardiac muscle, which forces blood through the body as a result of the pumping action of the heart. Elasticity refers to the ability of a muscle to return to its original shape after being stretched. Extensibility is the ability of muscle to stretch beyond its original shape.

Skeletal muscles

Skeletal muscles are those which are striated and attached to the bones through tendons. When muscles constrict or expand, they exert a force on the tendon. The tendon pushes or pulls the bone, which causes the limb or appendage to move. Tendons are not as elastic as muscles, so the majority of the body's movement is due to muscles. Skeletal muscles are primarily voluntary. They do, however, possess some involuntary characteristics that can also cause the muscle to contract or expand. Massage focuses on a therapeutic regimen designed to enhance the function of muscles through techniques that bring about relaxation, release of toxins, greater flexibility, and a greater range of motion. All of these results are accomplished through specific, pressurized body movements.

Point of insertion

Muscles are connected by tendons that extend from either end of the muscle. In order for movement to occur, one side of the muscle, generally the part closest to the center of the body, is considered the point of origin. This area is not as flexible as the other end of the muscle because of the lack of space in the area, and also because a broader range of motion is not necessary in that area. At the other end of the muscle lies the insertion point. This area is more distal, and the majority of the movement takes place here. Both the origin and the insertion point of the muscle are attached to the bone by a tendon. When one knows the origin of the muscle, it is easy to infer which way the muscle will contract based on that knowledge.

Actions of muscles

Although muscles are distinct within the body, they work in conjunction with other muscles to perform actions. As such, the muscle performing the primary movement is known as the prime mover, or the agonist. To counteract this initial movement, a muscle on the opposite side causes an opposite reaction. This muscle is known as the antagonist. For example, a bicep that contracts would be the agonist, while a triceps that expands would be classified as the antagonist. It is important to understand the relationship between the muscles so an appropriate treatment plan that takes the movement of both muscles into consideration can be created. Any muscles that assist the prime mover are called synergists. A fixator is any muscle that helps to stabilize a body part so another muscle can move.

Major Muscles

Trapezius muscle

The scapula is located on the posterior upper region of the body and connects the arm bone to the collarbone. The scapula is also known as the shoulder blade, while the collarbone is referred to as the clavicle. The trapezius muscle is connected to the cervical spine from the occipital bone at the top of the spine down to the T5-T12 area of the lumbar column. Three types of trapezius muscles exist: upper, middle, and lower. Each corresponds to the region in which the muscles originate. These muscles are involved with the elevation, depression, and upward rotation of the scapula.

Rhomboid muscle

There are major and minor components of the rhomboid muscle. The rhomboid major can be found in the T2-T5 portion of the thoracic vertebral column. It is located deep within the trapezius muscle. The purpose of the rhomboid major is to keep the scapula in line with the ribcage. This muscle functions by pulling the scapula closer to the vertebral column. The rhomboid minor retracts the scapula downward. It is found between the C7-T1 vertebral column. Its point of insertion is at the base of the scapula.

Levator scapulae muscle

This muscle originates from the C1-4 vertebral column, which is located at the back and side of the neck. It helps to move the neck from side to side laterally. It inserts at the top third of the scapula.

Pectoralis minor muscle

This muscle originates between the 3rd and 5th ribs, close to the costal cartilage. The pectoralis minor draws the scapula downward and towards the thorax. It attaches on the coracoid process, which extends outward from the scapula.

Serratus anterior muscle

This muscle originates from anterior ribs 1-8 and causes an upward movement of the scapula. It provides stabilization and is also referred to as the "boxer's muscle" because it assists with protraction of the scapula.

Upper extremities muscle

Approximately eight separate muscles cause the upper arm to move. These muscles are listed below:
- Pectoralis Major (Clavicular and Sternal): helps to push the shoulder forward and rotate the arm towards the body
- Coracobrachialis: helps the arm swing forward
- Deltoid (Anterior, Middle, and Posterior): mainly responsible for lifting the arm away from the trunk at the shoulder
- Supraspinatus: primarily involved in abduction of the shoulder
- Infraspinatus: helps to extend the arm and rotate it to the outside
- Subscapularis: involved in the medial rotation of the arm
- Teres minor: involved with the adduction and lateral rotation of the arm
- Teres major: involved with arm extension and medial rotation
- Latissimus Dorsi: the major muscle of the upper back, which assists in moving the arm backward and rotating it inward

Pectoralis major and coracobrachialis muscles

The pectoralis major is divided into two groups: the clavicular portion and the sternal portion. The clavicular portion originates medially at the clavicle and inserts at the outer ridge of the bicipital groove. Its causative actions are the conduction of adduction, the moving of the limb closer to the body, medial rotation, and flexion of the humerus bone. The humerus is the long bone extending from the scapula at the shoulder to the radius and ulna at the elbow. The sternal portion of the pectoralis major originates from the sternum and the costal cartilage of ribs 1-6, but inserts at the outer ridge of the bicipital groove proximally. It acts on the arm in the same manner and also causes the extension of the humerus when it is flexed. The coracobrachialis originates at the coracoid process of the scapula (the portion of the scapula that extends frontward), and inserts at the middle of the humerus. It assists with the flexion and adduction of the humerus bone.

Deltoid muscle

The deltoid is a triangular-shaped muscle that provides the rounded shape to the human shoulder. It is divided into three sections: anterior, middle, and posterior. The main motion associated with the deltoid is the abduction of the arm. The anterior section originates at the outside third of the clavicle. It inserts at the deltoid tuberosity of the humerus, and causes flexion and horizontal rotation of the humerus. The middle deltoid muscle originates at the acromion process of the scapula, and also inserts at the deltoid tuberosity. It assists with the adduction of the humerus to a 90-degree extension. The posterior deltoid originates at the lower part of the scapula and inserts at the deltoid tuberosity. It causes the extension, horizontal adduction, and lateral rotation of the humerus.

Supraspinatus muscle

This muscle originates at the supraspinous fossa of the scapula at the superior portion of this bone. Its insertion point is at the top of the humerus bone. This muscle acts upon the upper arm by instigating abduction in the humerus.

Infraspinatus muscle

This muscle originates at the infraspinous fossa of the scapula at the medial portion of this bone. It covers a much larger surface area than the supraspinous fossa. This muscle inserts at the greater tubercle, or large round nodule, of the humerus and assists in the lateral rotation of the humerus.

Subscapularis muscle

ANTERIOR

This muscle originates at the ~~back~~ surface of the scapula. This muscle inserts at the lesser tubercle of the humerus. Its function is to assist in the medial rotation of the humerus.

Teres major, teres minor, and latissimus dorsi muscles

EXT, IR, ADD ER   EXT, IR, ADD

The teres major is a thick, flat muscle located on the dorsal inferior side of the scapula. The insertion point is the lesser tubercle of the humerus. This muscle extends upward into the tubercle and is responsible for moving the humerus in a way that causes the arm ~~to lower~~ and move in a backward motion. The teres minor is a narrow, long muscle that is part of the rotator cuff. The insertion point is the lowest end of the greater tubercle of the humerus. It causes the humerus to move in a backward motion and also to rotate outward. The latissimus dorsi is a large, triangular, flat muscle located on the posterior side of the body. It covers the lumbar region and the last six of the thoracic vertebrae. This muscle extends upwards to insert at the intertubercular groove of the humerus. The actions it is responsible for are the extension, adduction, and internal rotation of the joint at the shoulder.

Biceps brachii muscle

The biceps brachii is the muscle located on the anterior upper arm. It is often referred to simply as the bicep. Its main purpose is to cause the flexion of the arm. The origin of the bicep is at the coracoid process of the scapula (short head) and the glenoid fossa (long head). It then extends down the arm and attaches at the radial tuberosity, a large nodule at the end of the radius. Because of the insertion point, the biceps brachii also influences the movement of the forearm.

Actions caused by the biceps brachii.
There are three actions caused by the biceps brachii: flexion of the forearm, extension of the arm above the shoulder joint, and the supination of the forearm (forearm rotation that results in the palms facing upwards). The triceps brachii is located on the posterior region of the upper arm. It originates at three points: the infraglenoid tuberosity of the scapula, the proximal half of the humerus, and the distal region of the humerus. The triceps brachii is responsible for extending the elbow. The biceps and triceps work in conjunction as flexors and extensors. The flexor contracts the muscle, causing the joint to bend, while the contraction of the extensor causes the limb to return to its original position.

Supinator muscle, pronator teres, and pronator quadratus

The supinator is a wide muscle that curves around the upper third of the radius. Its main purpose is to allow the hand and forearm to supinate, or twist, so that the palm of the hand either faces the body or faces forward. It also uses the bicep brachii muscle to perform this action. The supinator consists of two types of fibers: the superficial fibers and the upper fibers. This muscle can be difficult to palpate. The pronator teres and the pronator quadratus are two muscles that work together to pronate the hand so that the palm faces downwards towards the floor. The pronator teres originates at both the humerus and the ulna. It then attaches at the radius. The pronator quadratus runs from the distal part of the anterior ulna to the distal part of the anterior radius. This muscle assists not only with moving the palm to face downwards, but also with keeping the bones of the radius and ulna together.

26

Flexion of the wrist

The muscles that play a part in causing flexion of the wrist are:
- Flexor Carpi Radialis – This muscle can be felt on the anterior side of the forearm. It can be palpated on the radial side of the palmaris longus tendon; it helps to flex and abduct the hand.
- Flexor Carpi Ulnaris (humeral head and ulnar head) – This muscle is located on the proximal half of the forearm; it helps to flex and adduct the hand.
- Palmaris Longus – This muscle originates from the humerus and inserts at the palmar aponeurosis, also known as the muscles of the palm of the hand. Somewhat superfluous, this muscle assumes a more prominent role when other muscles are injured.

Extension of the wrist

The muscles that play a role in causing the extension of the wrist are:
- Extensor Carpi Radialis Longus – This muscle originates at the distal third of the humerus and inserts at the base of 2nd metacarpal or index finger. It moves the wrist in such a way that the hand is moved away from the palm and towards the thumb.
- Extensor Carpi Radialis Brevis – This muscle originates on the lateral side of the humerus and inserts at the base of the 3rd metacarpal, or middle finger. It holds the wrist in place during flexion of the fingers and aids in the adduction of the hand.
- Extensor Carpi Ulnaris – This muscle originates on the lateral humerus and inserts at the lateral base of the 5th metacarpal, or pinky finger; it extends and adducts the wrist.

Finger Muscles

The following is a partial list of the muscles that act upon the fingers:
- Flexor Digitorum Superficialis: (includes humeral head, ulnar head, and radial head); flexes the wrist, interphalangeal joints, and hand
- Flexor Digitorum Profundus: flexes the distal and proximal interphalangeal joints, metacarpophalangeal joints (except the thumb), and the hand
- Flexor Digiti Minimi: flexes the little finger
- Extensor Digitorum: extends the wrist and the fingers (except the thumb)
- Extensor Indicis: extends the metacarpophalangeal joint of the index finger
- Extensor Digiti Minimi: helps to extend the wrist and the fifth metacarpophalangeal joint

Muscles that act upon the fingers
The following is a partial list of the muscles that act upon the fingers:
- Adductor Digiti Minimi: abducts and flexes the fifth metacarpophalangeal joint
- Opponens Digiti Minimi: coordinates the movements of the little finger in relation to the thumb
- Palmar Interosseous: (includes first, second, third, and fourth); helps to flex and adduct the metacarpophalangeal joints
- Dorsal Interosseous: adducts the 2nd and 4th metacarpophalangeal joints, assists in radial and ulnar deviation of the 3rd metacarpophalangeal joint, and flexes the 2nd, 3rd, and 4th metacarpophalangeal joints
- Lumbricals: flexes the metacarpophalangeal joints and extends the interphalangeal joints

Thigh and lateral rotators muscles

The muscles of the lateral rotators and thigh are made up of the gluteus maximus, which provides for lateral movement and support of the thigh; the gluteus medius, which adducts the thigh; and the gluteus minimus, which assists with rotating the hip. The internal rotators include the quadratus femoris, the obturator externus and internus, and the gemellus superior and inferior. These muscles aid in rotating the hip area. Additional muscle groups include the adductor brevis, the adductor longus, and the adductor magnus. These muscles assist with the extension and rotation of the thigh. The psoas major and the iliacus are located in the pelvic region and assist with flexing the thigh and hip and rotating the knee.

Upper leg muscles

The posterior thigh region is composed of the biceps femoris, the semi-tendinosis, and the semi-membranous. These muscles assist with extending the thigh and rotating the knee. The biceps femoris is more commonly known as the hamstring, and is made up of the long head and the short head. The long head of the biceps femoris originates at the ischial tuberosity and the sacrotuberous ligament. It inserts on the lateral side of the fibula and the tibia. The short head originates at the lateral edge of the linea aspera, a rough ridge on the posterior portion of the fibula. Both of these help with the lateral rotation of the leg and hip. Other muscles that cause the leg to extend at the knee include the rectus femoris, vastus lateralis, vastus intermedius, and the vastus medialis.

Foot muscles

The following is a partial list of muscles that act on the foot and cause movement as a result of inversion, extension, and flexion:
- Popliteus: responsible for medial rotation and flexion of the leg below the knee
- Tibialis Anterior: responsible for dorsiflexion and inversion
- Peroneus Tertius: responsible for dorsiflexion and eversion; not present in all people
- Extensor Digitorum Longus: responsible for dorsiflexion and eversion of the foot as well as extension of the toes
- Extensor Hallucis Longus: responsible for dorsiflexion and inversion of the foot, as well as extension of the big toe

<u>Muscles that act on the foot</u>
The following is a partial list of muscles that act on the foot and cause movement as a result of inversion, extension, and flexion:
- Gastrocnemius (Medial Head and Lateral Head): responsible for flexing the knee during foot dorsiflexion and flexing the plantar during knee extension
- Plantaris: flexes the knee
- Soleus: responsible for plantar flexion
- Flexor Digitorum Longus: responsible for plantar flexion, inversion, and toe flexion
- Flexor Hallucis Longus: primarily responsible for plantar flexion, inversion, and toe flexion
- Tibialis Posterior: responsible for plantar flexion and inversion
- Peroneus Longus: responsible for eversion and plantar flexion
- Peroneus Brevis: responsible for eversion and plantar flexion

Abdominal region muscles

Several muscle groups act upon the abdominal area. These include the rectus abdominus, which is responsible for flexing the trunk and tensing the abdominal walls. The external obliques run alongside the external surfaces of the lower eight ribs. These muscles extend from below the armpit down towards the waist. They allow for bilateral movement and the side to side rotation of the trunk. The internal obliques lie just underneath the external, and provide for the same movements as the external obliques. The transverse abdominis muscles lie underneath the rectus abdominis, and also help with flexion and compression of the abdominal wall. The rectus abdominis can be palpitated from the sternum down to the pubis. The external obliques can be felt on the lateral side of the abdomen. The internal obliques and the transverse abdominis are situated deep within the abdominal region; they cannot be palpitated.

Respiratory process muscles

The primary muscle used to assist with the respiratory process is the diaphragm. It is located between the upper lumbar vertebrae and within the region of the six lowest ribs and costal cartilage. The diaphragm has no insertion point. The main purpose of the diaphragm is to contract the muscles used for inspiration (the intake of air). The muscle cannot be palpitated, but can be seen during the respiratory process. Other respiratory muscles include the intercostals, which are made up of the external, internal, and innermost components. These muscles are located between each of the ribs and serve to pull apart the ribs during inspiration, allowing for greater lung capacity. The serratus posterior superior, located near the collarbone, and the serratus posterior inferior, located at the base of the ribs, serve to expand the ribs outwards and downwards, which also leads to an increase in lung capacity.

Spinal column muscle

The following is a list of the muscles that run alongside the spinal column. All are difficult to palpitate through the skin.
* Quadratus Lumborum: responsible for lateral flexion of the spine
* Intertransversarii: located between the transverse processes of the vertebrae
* Interspinales: found in pairs located on either side of the contiguous vertebrae
* Rotatores: located only in the thoracic region; assists in flexion of the spine
* Multifidus: assists in the rotation of the spine
* Semispinalis: (includes capitis, cervicis, and thoracis); longitudinal muscles connected to the vertebrae
* Spinalis: (includes capitis, cervicis, and thoracis); bundled with a group of tendons and directly next to the spine
* Longissimus: (includes capitis, cervicis, and thoracis); help to extend the vertebral column, flex the spine laterally, and rotate the head and neck to either side

Muscles that aid in mastication

Mastication is defined as the act of chewing, which is the process by which the teeth break food down into smaller particles that are easily swallowed. Many muscles aid this process. The masseter is responsible for closing the jaw, and can be found near the zygomatic arch and the mandible. The temporalis, which originates at the temporal bone, causes the jaw to close and retract. The buccinator, which originates at the maxilla and mandible, helps to keep the cheeks close to the teeth to allow the food to remain in place for chewing. The internal pterygoid helps to close the jaw and move the jaw from side to side. The external pterygoid causes the lower jaw to protrude forward, an action associated most often with an under bite.

Eye muscles

The muscles of the eye provide for side-to-side and up-and-down movement. They allow a person to focus on objects without moving their head. None of these muscles can be palpitated. The eye muscles are as follows:
* Levator Palpebrae Superioris – Causes the eyelid to open
* Superior Oblique – Causes the eye to turn out and downwards
* Superior Rectus – Causes the eye to rotate upwards
* Lateral Rectus – Causes lateral movement
* Inferior Rectus – Moves the eye downwards
* Medial Rectus – Moves the eye medially
* Inferior Oblique – Moves the eye upwards and out

Facial muscles

The muscles that are used to form the facial expressions associated with happiness, sadness, anger, etc. are aided by the following muscle groups:
- Epicranius: (also known as the occipitofrontalis); runs from the occipital bone to the frontal bone; helps to raise the eyebrow
- Corrugator: lowers the medial end of the eyebrow and wrinkles the brow
- Procerus: originates from the membrane that covers the bridge of the nose; assists the motion of the frontal bone
- Orbicularis Oculi: lowers the eyelids
- Nasalis: compresses the cartilage of the nose
- Dilator Naris: helps to manipulate the nostrils
- Quadratus Labii Superioris: raises the upper lip
- Zygomaticus: moves the mouth up and back
- Orbicularis Oris: puckers the lips
- Risorius: brings the edges of the mouth backwards; associated with a smile or grimace
- Depressor Anguli Oris: lowers the angle of the mouth
- Depressor Labii Inferioris: lowers the lower lip
- Mentalis: responsible for movement of the mouth back and down; associated with a frown
- Platysma: draws the lower lip down, wrinkling the neck and upper chest
- Auricularis: wiggles the ears

Forehead muscles

The muscle groups that assist the body perform movements such as frowning, drawing the eyebrows together, wrinkling the forehead, and drawing the nose upwards are listed below:
- Epicranius (consisting of the occipitalis and frontalis) – This muscle originates just above the occipital ridge and inserts at the epicranial aponeurosis. This muscle draws the epicranius towards the back, or posterior, of the head. It also raises the eyebrows, which causes the forehead to wrinkle. This muscle is sometimes known as the occipitofrontalis.
- Corrugator – This muscle is also known as the corrugator supercilii. It is triangular in shape and is responsible for wrinkling the forehead and frowning.
- Procerus – The origin of this muscle is within the fascia over the cartilage in the nasal area. It inserts between the eyebrows and deep within the skin. This muscle is responsible for the action of wrinkling the nose.

Muscles that aid in the movement of the eyes and nostrils
The muscles that are involved with this region of the face include:
- Orbicularis Oculi – Controls the opening and closing of the eye. This muscle originates at the nasal bone and circles the eyeball. The insertion point of this muscle is all around the eye; the muscle blends in with the surrounding areas.
- Nasalis – This muscle originates above the incisors at the maxilla bone. It then blends in with the procerus muscle. The purposes of this muscle are to compress the bridge of the nostrils, allow the external area of the nostrils to elevate, or flare, and also to depress the tip of the nose.
- Dilator Naris – This muscle allows the nostril opening to expand. It originates at the greater alar cartridge and inserts at the end point of the nose.

Mouth muscles

There are about eight muscle groups that are responsible for the various movements of the mouth. They include:

- Quadratus Labii Superioris – This lies next to the nose and extends to the zygomatic arch. It is responsible for raising or elevating the upper lip.
- Zygomaticus (major and minor) – This muscle extends from one side of the zygomatic arch to the corner of the mouth. The contraction of this muscle causes the mouth to draw back and upwards; this movement is associated with smiling.
- Orbicularis Oris – This muscle originates from various muscles around the mouth and inserts at the lips. It is a circular muscle that allows the mouth to remain closed, aids in chewing, helps with speech, and aids in the formation of facial expressions.
- Risorius – This muscle originates over the masseter. It inserts at the muscle surrounding the mouth and at the corners of the mouth. It is responsible for moving the mouth backwards at an angle.
- Depressor Anguli Oris – This muscle is responsible for drawing the mouth into a downward position and is located at the outer edge of the chin.
- Depressor Labii Inferioris – This muscle helps to depress the lower lip.
- Mentalis – This muscle causes the chin to rise up and also enables a person to pout.
- Platysma – This muscle causes the mouth to move in a downward direction, enabling a person to form an expression of sadness. It also causes the skin of the neck to wrinkle.

Proprioception

Proprioception is the body's ability to gauge its own position in the external world. At all times, we are engaged in unconscious acts of proprioception that allow us to move around in harmony with our surroundings. Proprioception is often referred to as spatial orientation. Scientists believe that the human capacity for proprioception can be attributed to the endings of peripheral nerve fibers in the muscles and joints. The information that is obtained from these nerve endings is integrated with information from other sources, including the visual, auditory, tactile, and vestibular systems. The vestibular system senses the velocity of head movements and the relative pull of gravity on the body, and can therefore provide important information about the orientation of the body.

Muscle spasm

A muscle spasm is a dysfunction of the muscle in which involuntary contractions occur in a single muscle or a group of muscles. The intensity of these spasms can vary depending on the person's pain tolerance and how long the contractions continue. These spasms are classified as tonic when they remain in a contracted state for an extended time, and as clonic when the spasm relaxes between contractions. Another term for a muscle spasm is cramp. Typical kinds of spasms include hiccups, charley horses, twitches, and convulsions. Muscles can also spasm as a result of nearby injuries. When treating a spasm, massaging the area directly is not recommended until the acute spasm has subsided. It is thought that compressing the ends of the muscle or preventing the contraction of the antagonist muscles will help quiet the muscle spasm. Massaging the area after the acute phase has passed will help eliminate toxins from the muscle, introduce nutrients to the area, and restore circulation.

Muscle strains

The term muscle strains can also refer to torn or pulled muscles. There are generally three degrees of strains that can occur to the muscle. A grade 1 strain is when the muscle fibers have been overextended, but there are very few tears in the fibers. There is pain, but there are no visual marks on the surface of the skin. There is also no loss of muscle function. When a grade 2 strain occurs, there are partial tears in less than 50% of the muscle fibers. There is pain, tenderness, inflammation, and loss of function to some degree. A grade 3 strain is when more than 50% of the muscle fibers are torn. There is considerable pain, and the bleeding may be seen under the skin. Swelling and immediate loss of muscle function occurs.

31

Recovering from these types of injuries usually involves the use of the R.I.C.E. method (rest, ice, compression, and elevation) and massage once the acute stage has passed. It is important to maintain a good range of motion and flexibility once this stage is over to prevent muscle atrophy and scarring.

Hypertrophy and atrophy

It is possible for muscles to increase in size and get larger. As seen in bodybuilders, the size of the muscle increases through repeated strength training. This increase in the width of a muscle is known as hypertrophy. The muscular fibers themselves do not increase in number. Rather, the width of the muscle fibers increases. This increase causes the body part affected by the muscle to grow stronger. It will have more power while performing required actions or movements. Other changes that occur are an increase in the blood supply to the hypertrophic muscle and also an increase in ATP and mitochondria. Muscle atrophy refers to the degeneration and wasting away of muscles, which occurs as a result of disuse. Muscles that are not used break down and shrink, gradually losing their strength. The amount of blood supplied to the limb decreases, causing a change in the color of the limb. Atrophy commonly occurs in individuals with paralysis who have lost nerve connections to the muscles, which causes them to waste away.

Joints

The body has several different types of joint to allow for different kinds of movement. In a ball-and-socket joint, one of the connecting surfaces is rounded and the other is concave. As with all joints, a ball-and-socket joint is filled with fluid to allow for the smooth movement of the two parts. In a hinge joint, the convex surface of one joint fits against the concave surface of the other, and is arranged such that motion can only occur in one plane. An elbow is an example of a hinge joint. In a gliding joint, both connecting surfaces are basically flat, and so movement is very limited. The intercarpal joints connecting the mass of bones at the base of the hand is an example of a gliding joint.

Types of joints

In an ellipsoid joint, the oval-shaped section of one bone fits into the elliptical cavity of another. This connection allows for movement in two planes. The wrist is a classic example of an ellipsoid joint. In a pivot joint, a pointed or rounded area in one bone fits into a ring-like structure in another. In a joint like this, in the joint connecting the base of the spine and pelvis for example, the joint can only move by rotating. In a saddle joint, both of the connecting surfaces are shaped like saddles and fit together snugly. In this type of joint, movement can occur in two planes. The best example of a saddle joint is the one which connects the thumb to the hand.

Joint capsules

A joint capsule is a sort of sleeve that surrounds a joint, preventing any loss of fluid and binding together the ends of the bones in the joint. The outside of this sleeve is made of a tough material, while the inside is softer and looser. In this way, movement is not impeded. Joint capsules are often especially stringy in areas where movement should be discouraged. For instance, there is a strong joint capsule section on the back of the knee, which is one reason why it is difficult for the lower leg to bend forward. The fibers of the outer joint capsule are known as ligaments; the inside of the joint capsule is called the synovial membrane. The synovial membrane secretes a fluid that keeps the joint lubricated and removes debris.

Ranges of motion

When describing the range of motion of a joint, massage therapists distinguish between the active, passive, and resistant ranges of motion. The active range of motion is the amount of flexibility the client is able to achieve without any external aid. The passive range of motion, on the other hand, is the degree of flexibility that can be achieved through the massage therapist's manipulations; no effort is expended by the client. Finally, the resistant range of motion is the degree of flexibility that can be achieved when the joint is acting against some form of resistance. For instance, a resistant range of motion assessment might measure the degree of flexibility of the elbow during a biceps curl.

Effects of diseases on muscular system

Tendonitis, tenosynovitis, and lupus

Tendonitis is the condition in which the tendon that connects the muscle to the bone becomes inflamed. Tenosynovitis is the inflammation that occurs along the tendon sheath. Both of these conditions cause pain, stiffness, and swelling of the affected area. Treatment regimens include massage over the inflamed area, the application of ice to decrease swelling, and physical manipulation to increase range of motion and assist with prevention of scar tissue. Lupus is an autoimmune disease that can affect tissues and organs. This disease affects the connective tissue and can cause pain throughout many areas of the body. With this disease, blood vessels may become inflamed and arthritis can occur. Massage therapy on a person with lupus should be performed under the supervision of a physician to prevent pain to the patient.

Fibromyalgia and muscular dystrophy

Fibromyalgia is a disease that also affects connective tissue, producing pain, stiffness, and fatigue in the muscles, tendons, and ligaments. Factors such as temperature, humidity, and infections can cause an increase in the person's discomfort level and trigger additional symptoms. With the pain levels of each person varying, it is important to work with the client's personal physician to develop a massage plan. Muscular dystrophy is a disease that causes progressive degeneration of the muscles in the body. The muscular fibers are gradually replaced by fat and connective tissues, eventually leaving the muscle unable to function. If it does not induce pain, massage is beneficial in preventing the onset of muscle degeneration.

Pathologies and Massage Therapy

Common pathologies

The effects of massage therapy on many common pathologies are as follows:
- Asthma: tightening of the bronchial tubes; results in wheezing, coughing, and trouble breathing; massage can help to strengthen the muscles involved in breathing
- Chronic bronchitis: inflammation and infection of the bronchi; often occurs in conjunction with emphysema; massage can be helpful, so long as the patient is monitored closely
- Pneumonia: inflammation of the lungs; manifests as fever, chills, chest pain, cough, and difficulty breathing; massage is beneficial once the patient has passed out of the acute phase
- Cold: viral infection of the upper respiratory tract; symptoms can include fever, coughing, mucus overproduction, and headache; massage is helpful for managing symptoms and strengthening the immune system
- Atherosclerosis: hardening of the arteries; individuals with this condition should not receive rigorous circulatory massage
- Thrombus: a blood clot that remains fixed in the blood stream; massage is contraindicated
- Embolism: a blood clot that is moving through the bloodstream; massage is contraindicated
- Emphysema: hardening of the alveoli in the lungs; symptoms include trouble breathing, cough, and chronic respiratory infection; massage can be performed if the patient can breathe effectively and the condition is not acute
- Hypertension: high blood pressure in the pulmonary arteries; massage is indicated if the individual is not suffering from kidney or cardiovascular conditions
- Benign prostatic hyperplasia: irregular growth of the prostate gland; may cause problems with urination; does not prevent massage
- Endometriosis: overgrowth of endometrial cells in the peritoneal cavity; may lead to heavy menstruation, abdominal pain, and problems with intercourse and/or evacuation; massage is indicated, except in the affected area
- Peritonitis: inflammation of the membrane along the inner wall of the abdomen and pelvis; caused by infection or disease; manifests in severe abdominal pain; massage is contraindicated and the client should receive immediate medical attention
- Prostatitis: inflammation of the prostate gland; may result in chills, fever, testicular pain, pain in the lower back, and difficulty with urination; circulatory massage is contraindicated if the patient is in the acute phase
- Boils: bacterial infections on the skin; manifests as red sores; often appear in clusters; should not be massaged, especially because they may be quite contagious
- Bunions: a growth of the bone at the base of the big toe; should not be massaged
- Burns: may be first-degree (slight inflammation), second-degree (damage to epidermis), or third-degree (including damage to the dermis); once the burn has passed out of the acute stage, it may be massaged so long as it does not hurt
- Bedsores: lesions caused by impaired circulation; should not be massaged directly, although massage is a good way to prevent bedsores
- Fungal infections: manifest on the skin as red, itchy patches and blisters; may result in the weakening and infection of finger and toe nails; massage is contraindicated at the site of the infection
- Herpes: a virus that causes lesions and blisters; contraindicated in the acute stage and when the client has an infection or outbreak; equipment that comes into contact with the client should be washed
- Hives: a raised, scratchy patch of skin; usually caused by an allergic reaction; during the acute phase, massage is contraindicated everywhere; after the acute phase passes, massage is only contraindicated in the area of the hives
- Lice: parasitic insects; most often found on the scalp; symptoms include itching, irritation, and sores; massage is contraindicated, especially because lice are highly contagious

- HIV/AIDS: a disease that ravages the immune system; HIV becomes AIDS when it integrates into the DNA of the individual; massage is indicated so long as the client is in relatively good health
- Cystic fibrosis: disease which results in exceptionally thick production of mucus, sweat, bile, and other body products; symptoms may include problems with breathing, coughing, and lung infections; massage is indicated, unless the patient's symptoms preclude it
- Cancer: a growth of malignant cells; massage can be beneficial so long as it does not reduce the body's strength during a period of intense and debilitating treatments
- Multiple sclerosis: a permanent disease; manifests in symptoms like numbness, blindness, and paralysis; massage is indicated in the subacute phase
- Depression: any diminution in quality of life, outlook, or happiness; massage can be extremely beneficial in mitigating the effects of depression
- Headaches: massage is indicated unless the headache is due to infection or damage to the central nervous system
- Premenstrual syndrome: a set of physical and psychological changes that occur directly before menstruation; symptoms can include breast tenderness, bloating, moodiness, and anger; bodywork can be especially beneficial while a woman is experiencing PMS
- Fever: slight increase in body temperature; massage is contraindicated; if a fever is greater than 102 degrees, the client should receive immediate physical attention
- Varicose veins: enlarged and twisted veins; may result in cramps and trouble with movement; massage is contraindicated locally
- Warts: small growths on the outer layer of skin; contracted by contact with another wart; massage is contraindicated locally
- Cysts: pockets of connective tissue surrounding a foreign body; should not be massaged directly
- Lyme disease: an inflammatory disease caused by a bacterium transmitted by deer ticks; can result in a rash, symptoms of influenza, and pain in the joints; massage can improve joint function during subacute phases
- Cerebral palsy: a family of injuries to the central nervous system; symptoms may include poor coordination, involuntary movements, and muscular disfiguration; massage can be very beneficial for individuals with cerebral palsy
- Meningitis: an inflammation of the membranes that surround the brain and spinal cord; can be caused by bacteria, protozoa, or viruses; massage is strictly contraindicated during the acute phase; once this passes massage can be beneficial
- Muscular dystrophy: a genetic disease in which the skeletal muscles gradually degenerate; may result in weakness, disability, and an inability to walk; massage can be quite effective at loosening muscles and improving circulation
- Bursitis: inflammation in the areas where tendons, ligaments, and bones come into contact; when acute, massage is contraindicated; otherwise, there is no restriction on massage
- Carpal tunnel syndrome: irritation of the nerves in the hands; often caused by repetitive tasks; massage may be beneficial, especially around the wrist area
- Encephalitis: swelling of the brain; caused by infection; symptoms include fever, headache, and disorientation; massage only contraindicated if the condition is acute
- Parkinson's disease: degenerative neurological disease; manifests in expressionless face, involuntary movements, tremor, and muscle weakness; massage is indicated, so long as the movements of the client are respected
- Heart attack: flow of blood through the heart is suddenly impeded; circulatory massage contraindicated during the recovery period
- Heart failure: heart is unable to supply enough blood to nourish the body; symptoms include lung fluid buildup, irregular pulse, and coughing; energetic massage is appropriate, but circulatory massage is strictly contraindicated
- Stroke: rapid death of brain cells; caused by a blockage of blood flow to the brain, which in turn results in an oxygen deficit; symptoms include loss of speech, weakness, and paralysis; all but the most vigorous circulatory massage is indicated for this group
- Gout: inflammation of the ankle and foot joints; feet and ankles will become swollen and painful; massage contraindicated

- Edema: build-up of fluid between the organs; manifests in bloated areas on the body; in a severe, "pitting" edema, the body will not return to its natural form when pressure is applied; massage is contraindicated
- Gallstones: crystals made of hardened bile or cholesterol; massage indicated unless the client is in severe pain
- Scarification: build up of scar tissue, as for instance over a wound; massage is contraindicated during the acute period
- Pancreatitis: inflammation of the pancreas; often caused by alcoholism or gallstones; symptoms include abdominal pain, nausea, vomiting, and fever; massage is appropriate once the condition has been thoroughly treated by a doctor
- Hernia: small tear in the abdominal lining or inguinal ring; small intestine may poke through this hole; massage is contraindicated until the hernia has been treated
- Irritable bowel syndrome: an intestinal disorder in which the bowels and their nerves become over or under active; can manifest in abdominal pain, bloating, diarrhea, and constipation; massage is indicated; client should be monitored
- Tuberculosis: contagious infection; can only be identified by a chest x-ray.
- Hepatitis: viral infection of the liver; massage is contraindicated when the disease is acute
- Diabetes: disorders of the metabolism; manifests in problems with appetite, urination, and blood sugar balance; massage is indicated unless the patient has specific circulation problems
- Hemophilia: condition in which the blood fails to clot normally; vigorous massage is contraindicated, though gentle techniques may be beneficial
- Hypoglycemia: low blood sugar; can manifest in anxiety, palpitations, sweating, and nausea; this condition is episodic, so if an individual is experiencing a bout of hypoglycemia, he or she should receive treatment before a massage
- Lupus: a disease in which chronic inflammation leads to degeneration of the immune system; can manifest in diseases of the skin, heart, lungs, kidneys, joints, and nervous system; massage is indicated so long as the client is not experiencing an acute episode
- Herniated disc: the matter between the vertebral discs is forced out, which puts pressure on the spinal cord and nerves; massage is indicated, so long as the condition is not acute
- Fractures: cracked or broken bones; massage contraindicated in the area of the fracture, though it can be beneficial elsewhere
- Osteoarthritis: gradual inflammation, disintegration, and loss of the joint cartilage; most often affects the feet, hands, spine, hips, and knees; during acute inflammation, massage is strictly contraindicated
- Osteoporosis: reduction in bone mass; leads to a greater frequency of fracture; massage is indicated so long as the client is not in any great pain
- Urinary tract infection: infection of the kidney, ureter, bladder, or urethra; symptoms may include painful urination and abdominal pain; circulatory massage is contraindicated during the acute phase; massage in the lower abdomen is contraindicated during the subacute phase
- Hyperthyroidism: excessive thyroid hormone production; can result in high heart rate, weight loss, and depression; massage can be beneficial, as it can reduce stress
- Hypothyroidism: deficiency of thyroid hormone; can result in fatigue, constipation, and weight gain; massage is indicated if it does not aggravate any accompanying atherosclerosis
- Renal failure: failure of the kidneys; may result in jaundice, edema, and even death; massage is systemically contraindicated during the acute and chronic phases
- Influenza: virus of the respiratory tract; can result in fever, loss of appetite, and weakness; massage is only appropriate if the influenza has passed out of the acute phase
- Mononucleosis: a chronic infection; can last for one or two months; symptoms include fever, fatigue, sore throat, and swollen lymph nodes; massage is contraindicated during the acute phase
- Myasthenia gravis: an autoimmune neuromuscular disorder; manifests in extreme muscular fatigue; massage is indicated, though it will not improve the condition in any significant way

- Spina bifida: a birth defect in which part of the spine remains exposed; may result in incontinence, limited mobility, and learning difficulties; massage is indicated as part of a comprehensive physical therapy program
- Menopause: the end of a woman's menstrual periods; usually diagnosed when a woman has not menstruated for one year; some related symptoms include mood swings, hot flashes, and fatigue; massage is extremely useful during menopause
- Recovery from surgery: the client should receive permission from his or her physician before receiving massage treatment
- Hematoma: deep intramuscular bruising; may or may not be visible externally; massage is contraindicated for acute hematoma; sub-acute hematoma may benefit from gentle circulatory massage
- Tremor: unnatural, repetitive shaking of the body; may be caused by illness, medication, or fear; massage is indicated
- Moles: pigmented spots on the skin; moles should not affect the delivery of massage services; however, moles that change in color or shape should be reported to the client's doctor
- Psoriasis: a red, scaly skin rash; most often located on the elbows, knees, and scalp; not contagious; contraindicated locally during the acute phase; indicated during the subacute phase
- Ulcers: any lesion that is eroding the membrane or surrounding skin; massage is contraindicated locally
- Tendinitis: inflammation of a tendon; usually caused by injury; massage is indicated, especially for reducing inflammation
- Plantar fasciitis: inflammation of the tissue that stretches from the heel to the ball of the foot; symptoms include pain and difficulty walking; massage is indicated, as it can delay the formation of scar tissue and improve circulation in the calves
- Shin splints: inflammation of the tibia; results from overuse; manifests in pain; massage is indicated so long as the client does not have a stress fracture
- Muscle spasms: short, involuntary muscle contractions; caused by stress, medication, and overuse; massage around the muscle connector sites can improve the condition and reduce painful symptoms

Herniated disk

A herniated disk is an invertebral disk that has protruded out and into the spinal cavity, causing pain and increased pressure on the spinal cord. This disk can also cause pain and radiating pressure on the nerve endings leading down the legs. Most often occurring in the lumbar region, the typical herniated disk occurs gradually over time. When seeing a physician for this condition, diagnostic tests may be ordered to determine the degree of severity. These tests can include x-ray, myelogram, CT scan, and MRI to determine the exact cause of the pain; the symptoms can mimic other illnesses or diseases. Initial treatment of a herniated disk includes hot or cold therapy, massage, exercise, stretching, rest, pain medication, and, in severe or prolonged cases, surgery.

Strain and sprain

Strains and sprains are two of the most common muscular injuries. They may be severe and painful, or so minor as to be almost unnoticeable. A strain is an injury that occurs when a muscle has been stretched beyond its capabilities. It can also be referred to as a pulled muscle. Microscopic tears within the muscle cause pain, stiffness, swelling, and sometimes bruising. A sprain is an injury that occurs when a ligament is overstretched suddenly, causing pain, immediate swelling, and bruising. Severe sprains involve a popping, either felt or heard, and loss of function of that body part.

Classifications of sprains
There are three main classifications of sprains. The first is identified as a class I sprain. This is when the ligament has been stretched, but there is little to no loss of limb function. The second is a class II sprain. The ligament is torn, and there is some loss of limb function. Some internal bleeding may occur, or there may not be any bruising or discoloration. The third type, a class III sprain, involves a complete tear of the

ligament, along with internal bleeding and extensive loss of function of the affected limb. All three types of sprains heal best when the R.I.C.E. method (rest, ice, compression, and elevation) is used. Massage is recommended only during the latent stages of healing and will help prevent the formation of scars and increase range of motion and flexibility.

Infections

An infection within the body is an indication of the presence of microorganisms (such as bacteria, fungi, parasites, and viruses) that are capable of causing harm to the body. These microorganisms generally enter the body through cuts in the skin, through nasal passages, or by coming into contact with the bodily fluids of other individuals. The damage infections cause can range from simple, localized illnesses to diseases that ravage the entire body. Local infections are those that affect one small area of the body. If the infection has spread to other areas or all over the body, it is termed a systemic infection.

Inflammation

It is important that massage techniques are not performed on localized areas that are infected or, in cases of systemic infection, on any part of the body. Inflammation can result from an infection and causes five major changes to the body: redness, heat, swelling, pain, and loss of all or some function of the affected body part. Inflammation is an indicator of tissue damage. It is the result of an inflow of blood to the area and an increase in the production of white blood cells to aid in the healing process. It is important that these areas are not massaged while inflammation is present or while the patient has a fever.

Contraindications to massage

When performing a massage on a new client, it is important that the therapist obtain as thorough a medical history as possible. A contraindication is any procedure or treatment plan that, for the sake of the client's benefit and well-being, is not advisable. There are three types of contraindications that can exist: absolute, regional, or conditional. An absolute contraindication indicates that a massage should not be performed under any circumstances. Examples of this would include shock, pneumonia, and pregnancy-related toxemia. A regional contraindication exists when a client cannot have massage performed on a specific region of the body due to injuries, such as open wounds; contagious conditions that could cause harm to the therapist; or other conditions like arthritis. In the latter case, massage would result in additional pain to the client if the affected areas were massaged. The final type of contraindication is conditional. This means that the massage therapist must make accommodations in the therapeutic plan to help the client obtain the most benefit from the massage, while avoiding the areas that could cause discomfort.

Massage on cancer patients

When performing a massage, the client's well-being is of the utmost importance. As such, the therapist should be aware of the contraindications of performing massage on a cancer patient.

A complete medical history should be taken, and the physician or oncologist should be consulted to determine if massage is a recommended and suitable form of treatment.
Factors to consider are:
- Location and type of cancer
- Stage of the cancer
- Additional sites for metastasis
- Treatment level of the cancer
- Immune system condition of the person at the time of the massage
- Stamina level and attitude of the person

During the actual massage, light or moderate pressure should be used. Areas where tumors are known to exist should not be subjected to deep massage.

Special Populations

Stress and pain during pregnancy

During a normal pregnancy, the mother can benefit from a massage, which will aid in decreasing the discomfort and aches associated with the back pain, leg pain, stress, and fatigue that occur during pregnancy. In order to provide the best care for the mother, it is important to note the mother's condition and to absolutely avoid massage when there is a risk of toxemia or pre-eclampsia. Massage is not an ideal way to address the high blood pressure, edema, nausea, and diarrhea associated with these conditions. Furthermore, massage can actually do harm to the mother. To prep the client, the massage therapist must ensure that both the mother and unborn child are in a comfortable position on the table, preferably facing up and in a semi-reclined position. If the client is lying on her side, it is important to place pillows under the head and between the knees to help support the back. Avoiding massage in the abdominal area is indicated. In addition, the therapist should not have the mother lie prone on her abdomen if she is in the latter stages of pregnancy.

Prenatal massage

While pregnancy is generally considered a happy time in a woman's life, it can bring about many physical changes that cause additional strain and stress on the body. These physical changes include a shifting of the joints to accommodate weight gain and the stretching of the ligaments to prepare the body for delivery. Some of these changes are due to hormones, and they can cause a pregnant woman to feel additional strain, which can only be relieved through rest and relaxation. The areas that are most often subjected to stresses during pregnancy include the neck, back, hips, legs, and feet. During massage, supporting cushions and bolsters can increase the comfort level of the mother and allow her to fully enjoy the benefits of massage. These benefits include inducing a relaxed state, improving the body's circulation, and soothing the nerves. The most common positions for the mother during massage include lying in the side-lying position and, during the earliest parts of the pregnancy, lying in the prone position.

Contraindications for prenatal massage

It is advised that massage therapy be performed in the prone position only during the first trimester, before the new mother is "showing." Reducing the time spent in this position helps to keep the fetus safe. At no time should prenatal massage be performed on the abdominal area. If the mother indicates problems with nausea, vomiting, diarrhea, or unusual vaginal discharge, massage should be withheld until the physician has been notified. In addition, if there is high blood pressure, lack of fetal movement, severe edema, or any abdominal pain, the mother should be referred to her physician immediately, as these symptoms can indicate a severe condition like toxemia or pre-eclampsia. A less serious condition to be aware of during prenatal massage would be the presence of varicose veins. Light effleurage may be performed in these areas, but moderate to heavy massage techniques should be avoided.

Infants

There is no reason why infants cannot receive as many positive benefits from massage as adults. There are some special considerations, however, when administering massage treatments to an infant. The duration of an infant massage is typically shorter, usually lasting about 15 minutes. Because infants cannot express themselves verbally, the massage therapist needs to be especially sensitive to signs of discomfort. It is best to use natural oil for lubrication. An infant massage usually starts with a client in the supine position. While in this position, the face, torso, arms, legs, and feet can be massaged. Effleurage, pétrissage, and tapotement can all be used during an infant massage. After a while, the infant can be placed into the prone position so that the back and neck can be massaged.

Elderly clients

Elderly individuals can receive many benefits from massage. Their skin and bones, however, may be more sensitive to stress and strain, so the massage therapist needs to be especially gentle when dealing with an elderly client. Also, elderly clients are more likely to be modest and may require more privacy when changing clothes. Elderly clients are likely to need special assistance while mounting and dismounting the massage table. Massage is contraindicated in elderly individuals with varicose veins, blood clots, or bedsores. At times, the improved circulation generated by massage therapy can confuse or disorient elderly clients, so the massage therapist needs to be especially sensitive to any signs of distress.

Disabled clients

Massage can be extremely beneficial for disabled individuals, so long as proper precautions are taken. Obviously, the precise precautions will depend on the disability. Individuals with sensory impairment, deafness or blindness for example, can receive normal massage therapy, though the therapist needs to be especially careful to clearly explain the success of the elements of the treatment. Clients who are on crutches are likely to have excessive strain on their triceps and wrists, while clients using wheelchairs are likely to have excessive tension in the muscles of the upper arm and back. When dealing with a paralyzed client, be sure to use gentle pressure, as the client will not be able to indicate injurious amounts of stress.

Pharmacology

Pharmacology is the study of the effects that drugs have on living organisms. With a large number of individuals on prescription therapy, it may be common for the massage practitioner to encounter someone who is on drug therapy, but also needs the services of a massage therapist. Medications can cause side effects that, if not made known to the massage practitioner, will continue in spite of treatment. As an example, some medications cause muscle pain and weakness. When the therapist is knowledgeable about the types of medications a client is taking, he or she can then adapt the massage sessions to avoid certain areas. Additionally, some medications may provide the same benefits as those obtained by massage. In these cases, the individual may see a decreased need for medication due to the relief obtained through massage. Part of the initial consultation should involve taking an inventory of the medications, supplements, vitamins, and herbs the client is taking.

Anti-anxiety drugs

Anti-anxiety drugs influence the central nervous system and calm an individual's violent reaction to stress. There are two classes of anti-anxiety drugs:
- Benzodiazepines: act by reducing the activity of the neurons in the brain; common brands include Halcion, Valium, Xanax, and Ativan; during massage, the client is at risk of entering a deep parasympathetic state, and should be monitored for dizziness
- Buspirone HCl: acts by reducing the uptake of dopamine and serotonin in the brain; sold under the brand name BuSpar; the client should receive extra stimulation during massage, as the nervous system may be suppressed

Antidepressants

Antidepressant medications alter the chemistry of the brain in order to alleviate the symptoms of depression. These drugs often take up to a month of use before yielding any positive results. There are three major classes of antidepressants, along with some other miscellaneous medications:

- Tricyclics: act by influencing the production of norepinephrine, serotonin, and acetylcholine; common brands include Tofranil, Elavil, and Norpramin; may result in dizziness during massage
- Monoamine oxidase inhibitors: act by limiting the activity of monoamine oxidase; common brands include Marplan and Nardate; sleepiness and dizziness may result from massage
- Selective serotonin reuptake inhibitors: act by managing the neurotransmitter serotonin; common brands include Prozac, Zoloft, Lexapro, Paxil, and Celexa; massage can occasionally lead to nausea or abdominal pain
- Miscellaneous anti-depressants: common brands include Effexor, Wellbutrin, and Serzone

Anti-inflammatories and analgesics

These medications are typically prescribed for individuals suffering from muscle pain. For this reason, massage therapists should be careful not to unwittingly injure a patient whose pain threshold is lower than normal. There are five classes of anti-inflammatories and analgesics:

- Salicylates: reduce fever and sensitivity to pain; common brands include Aspirin and Doan's Aspirin; vigorous massage should be avoided
- Acetaminophen: reduces pain and fever, but does not reduce inflammation; may be combined with caffeine or barbiturates; common brands include Tylenol and Anacin; massage should be gentle
- Nonsteroidal anti-inflammatory drugs: reduce inflammation and pain; common brands include Celebrex, Advil, Excedrin, Nuprin, and Aleve; watch out for abdominal bleeding and nausea
- Steroidal anti-inflammatory drugs: reduce inflammation, pain, and edema; common brands include Cortisone, Prednisol, and Decadron; deep-tissue massage should not be performed on clients who have been taking these drugs for a long time
- Opioids, mixed opioids: common brands include Codeine, OxyContin, Percocet, Darvon, Vicodin, and Demerol; morphine is also an opioid; massage should not include deep-tissue work, and the therapist should monitor the client's responsiveness

Autonomic nervous system disorder medications

These drugs are designed to treat conditions affecting the sympathetic and parasympathetic nervous systems. There are four classes of autonomic nervous system disorder medications:

- Cholinergics: act in a manner similar to the parasympathetic nervous system; common brands include Urecholine and Carbastat; massage should be gentle and the client should be monitored for responsiveness
- Anticholinergics: these drugs either stimulate or suppress particular organs or parts of the nervous system; common brands include Atropine, Ditropan, and Anaspaz; massage should be performed with the particular action of the drug taken into consideration
- Adrenergic drugs: act by stimulating the sympathetic nervous system; common brands include Dopamine, Epinephrine, and Albuterol; it may take longer to induce a parasympathetic response from a client taking this kind of medication
- Adrenergic blockers: hinder the action of the sympathetic nervous system; common brands include Flomax, Migranal, and Cardura; it will be easy for the client to enter a deep parasympathetic state

Cardiovascular drugs

Calcium channel blockers, and ACE inhibitors
Cardiovascular drugs either expand blood vessels or decrease the response of the sympathetic nervous system, thereby reducing the amount of stress placed on the heart. There are seven major classes of cardiovascular drugs:

- Beta blockers: act by reducing the impact of the sympathetic nervous system on the heart; common brands include Inderal, Normodyne, and Levatol; blood pressure should be monitored during massage
- Calcium channel blockers: expand the blood vessels; common brands include Norvasc, Cardene, and Isoptin; clients may suffer from dizziness, low blood pressure, and flushing
- ACE inhibitors: increase evacuation of water and sodium; common brands include Lotensin, Captopril, and Vasotec; may result in extremely low blood pressure

Digitalis, antilipemic drugs, diuretics, and antianginal medication

- Digitalis: strengthens and improves the efficiency of the heart; common brands include Digitek and Lanoxin; circulatory massage should be avoided
- Antilipemic drugs: reduce the amount of cholesterol in the blood; common brands include Questran, Lopid, Zocor, and Crestor; constipation and cramping are two common concerns that should be considered before the initiation of massage therapy
- Diuretics: increases the amount of urine created by the kidneys; common brands include Lasix, Bumex, Thalitone, and Lozol; care should be take to avoid stressing the kidneys or reducing the blood pressure to a dangerous level
- Antianginal medications: either increase the amount of oxygen sent to the heart or reduce the heart's need for oxygen; common brands include Cedocard, Monoket, Nitrostat, and Nitro-Glycerin; the massage should be stopped immediately if hypotension, dizziness, or cramping occur

Cancer drugs

Cancer drugs are administered to kill or stop the production of cancer cells. Remember that these drugs act by more or less attacking all the cells of the body, and clients will therefore be severely debilitated. For this reason, extreme care should be taken during massage therapy. There are six major classes of cancer drugs:

- Alkylating drugs: common types include nitrogen mustards, ethylamines, alkyl sulfonates, triazenes, piperazines, and nitrosoureas
- Antimetabolite drugs: common brands include Cladribine, Aminopterin, and Cytarabine
- Antineoplastics: can be antibiotic, hormonal, natural, or other; these drugs inhibit the growth and development of malignant cells

Clot management drugs

Clot management drugs manage the body's ability to stop bleeding. In a normal body, blood clots are formed from a combination of red blood cells, white blood cells, and platelets. There are two classes of clot management drugs:

- Anticoagulants: encourage the liver to produce chemicals that limit the formation of new blood clots; common brands include Heparin and Lovenox; clients on this medication may be susceptible to bruising
- Antiplatelet drugs: act by preventing platelets in the blood from congregating at potential clot sites; common brands include Aspirin, Pletal, and Empirin; clients may be especially susceptible to bruising

Diabetes management drugs

The number of people taking diabetes management medications is steadily increasing in the United States. A massage therapist must monitor the client closely during massage, as a sudden decrease in blood glucose levels has the potential to induce a hypoglycemic episode. There are two classes of diabetes management drugs:

- Insulin: enables the body to obtain energy from glucose in the blood; common brands include Humulin, Lantus, and Novolin; the injection area should be avoided during massage, and, if possible, clients should receive massage towards the beginning of their insulin cycle
- Oral glucose management drugs: reduce the production of sugar in the liver and increase the production of insulin in the pancreas; common brands include Diabinese, Glucotrol, Lucophage, and Precose; clients are at an increased risk of experiencing a hypoglycemic episode when taking this kind of medication

Muscle relaxants

Muscle relaxants reduce the amount of tension in muscular tissue. For this reason, it is especially important for massage therapists to be restrained in the amount of force they use during bodywork. These drugs are primarily prescribed to alleviate muscle spasms and the resulting pain. There are two classes of muscle relaxants:

- Centrally-acting skeletal muscle relaxants: act by depressing the central nervous system; common brands include Soma, Paraflex, Valium, Norflex, and Flexeril.
- Peripherally-acting skeletal muscle relaxants: act by diminishing the contractions of the muscles; commonly sold under the brand name Dantrium; stretching should not exceed the client's normal range of motion during massage.

Thyroid supplement drugs

Thyroid supplement medications are prescribed to treat hypothyroidism. There are three classes of thyroid supplement drugs:

- Levothyroxine sodium: imitate the natural secretions of the thyroid; common brands include Synthroid, Eltroxin, and Levoxyl; massage is indicated, and should not react with medications in any adverse way
- Desiccated extract: imitate the actions of the hormones produced by a healthy thyroid; common brands include Armour Thyroid, Nature-Thyroid, and Westhroid; no real effect on massage
- Liothyronine sodium: these drugs fulfill the same functions as other thyroid supplements and are generally only prescribed when the others are ineffective; common brands include Cytomel and Triostat; no negative interaction with massage

Definition of drug

Drugs are any chemical or herbal substances that are used to relieve the symptoms of an illness or disease. The term "drug" can also be used to refer to illegal substances that alter the mind's perception and the body's movement. Oftentimes, the drugs prescribed by a physician can produce adverse side effects on the human body that can interfere with any benefits obtained the drug. Some drugs have the ability to affect an entire system of the body, including drugs that affect the circulatory system. Some other drugs cause only a localized reaction, such as those used to alleviate the pain of a broken leg.

Classifying drugs

The federal Food and Drug Administration classifies drugs in order to protect the safety of the consumer. Drugs do not affect all individuals in the same manner, as a person's age, body weight, and height help to determine how fast the body absorbs the drug. Drugs are given a generic name when they are created by a pharmaceutical company. A specific trade name is then given to help consumers identify it and make it easier to remember. Drugs are classified according to their therapeutic abilities; thus, the same drug can fall under more than one classification.

Herbal supplements and vitamins

Herbal remedies have been around for many years, and their origins can be traced back to many cultural groups, including Native American and Chinese societies. Herbs have many uses, from cooking, to decoration, to healing. Depending on the purpose of the plant and the need for it, all parts may be used, from the flowers and seeds down to the roots. Compared to chemically-based drugs, herbs are more commonly prescribed by physicians in other parts of the world. Approximately 25% of all prescription drugs come from a natural botanical source, unlike other drugs that are chemically manufactured in a lab environment. People tend to purchase herbs and supplements as a means of preventing disease and maintaining good health, and as an additional form of treatment that is used in conjunction with standard pharmaceutical treatment methods. The massage therapist should have an understanding of the effects of herbal supplements because of their widespread use and because their effects could interact with prescription medications.

Physiological effects of massage

Western massage, otherwise known as Swedish massage, helps to relax the body, increase metabolism, speed healing, and provide emotional and physical relaxation. Similar massages on two individuals can produce two entirely different reactions. Techniques used in Swedish massage include light touches and gentle stimulation over the skin, which produce reflexive sensations. Mechanically stimulating the body by increasing pressure on the muscles and tissues results in an increase in blood flow to the area, causing an increase in nutrients and oxygen as well as the removal of wastes from the muscle. By the end of the massage session, the body is in a more relaxed state. There is an increase in flexibility and a decrease in pain. An increase in the production of sweat and oil from the glands can be seen by the end of the massage. There is an improvement in blood flow to the area, resulting in a temporary color change in the skin. Finally, the temperature of the skin increases.

Effects on muscular structure

When a massage is being performed, the muscles undergo a transformation that helps them increase their nutritional intake, improves circulation, and helps to stimulate cellular activity within the muscle. Massage relaxes tense muscles and helps to alleviate the pain associated with muscle spasms. During a massage, blood passes through the muscular tissue at a rate that is three times greater than when the muscle is at rest. This action brings new supplies of blood to the area, and assists with the removal of waste material. After strenuous exercise, massage helps to alleviate the pain, stiffness, and soreness associated with the exercise. If massage is prescribed as a therapy after an injury, there is less scarring and buildup of connective tissue in the muscles. Range of motion is also increased through massage. Circulation is also increased, which helps to reduce the time lost due to the injury.

Effects on nervous system

The nervous system is comprised of the central nervous system (made up of the brain and spinal cord) and the peripheral nervous system (made up of the autonomic nervous system, cranial nerves, and spinal nerves). The nervous system has the ability to be either stimulated or soothed, depending on the type of muscle massage being utilized. Techniques that stimulate the body include friction, percussion, and vibration. Light rubbing, rolling or wringing of the skin is known as the technique of friction. Percussion involves a series of tapping to increase the nervous irritability. Depending on the duration, percussion has the ability to numb the nerves within the area. Vibration involves applying shaking or trembling movements on the body part. The end result is the stimulation of peripheral nerves. Soothing techniques that produce a calming effect include light stroking of the skin and pétrissage, which are light, kneading movements on the skin. Putting pressure on a specific trigger point desensitizes the area and releases hypertension in the muscle.

Effects on autonomic nervous system

The autonomic nervous system is divided into two distinct areas: the sympathetic nervous system and the parasympathetic nervous system. The sympathetic nervous system is responsible for the "fight or flight" response, while the parasympathetic system counters these effects and helps to return the body to a relaxed state by reducing the heart rate and increasing circulation to bring about a relaxed state of being. The sympathetic nervous system, by contrast, increases the alertness of the body through the release of adrenaline and epinephrine. When a massage is performed, the reaction from the autonomic nervous system is initially one of invigoration, which gradually mellows into relaxation and sedation. The parasympathetic nervous system is stimulated, leading to a reduction in epinephrine, norepinephrine, and blood pressure.

Effects on circulatory system

When techniques such as massage, pressure, stroking, and percussion are performed on the body, the circulatory system responds in a favorable manner, which benefits the entire body. Stroking the skin lightly causes dilation in the capillaries. Applying stronger pressure while stroking leads to the skin taking on a flushed look and a longer-lasting period of dilation. Percussion of the muscles causes the blood vessels to contract; they gradually ease up and cause a relaxed state. Applying friction to the muscles and skin rapidly produces a response, in this case the flow of blood through the veins. It also accounts for the flow of interstitial fluid, which leads to a healthy cellular environment. Kneading the muscles causes the blood to flow into the deeper sections of arteries and veins. Lighter massage techniques are responsible for lymph circulation, as they diminish the tendency towards edema in these areas. Compression causes muscles to store a larger quantity of blood. Finally, all massage techniques should be directed towards the heart: from the ends of the appendages towards the torso and also from the head downward.

Pain relief

The massage therapist should pay close attention to areas of concern in the patient's body before, during, and after the massage. Techniques used during the massage have the ability to alleviate any suffering caused by pain or stress. Of particular interest to the therapist are methods that can relieve the pain of a pain-spasm-pain cycle, which is indicated by ischemia (decreased blood flow to the area within a muscle). A proper therapeutic massage increases blood flow to an area, creating pleasurable sensations where there was previously only marked pain. The nerve endings carry these signals to the brain, causing the overall feeling of calmness and relaxation throughout the body. To combat ischemia, the massage therapist should focus on breaking the pain-spasm-pain cycle and increasing mobility in that area. Through therapeutic palpations, the exact area of pain can be identified. The therapist can then focus the massage in that area, reduce the amount of lactic acid within the muscle, and introduce oxygen and other nutrients to help speed healing.

Pain management

Pain management is one of the benefits obtained through massage therapy, as the muscle receives an influx of blood circulating through the tissue. Through a process known as gate control theory, the transmission of pain sensations from the affected area is interrupted and prevented from reaching the central nervous system. This is accomplished through stimulating the cutaneous receptors. Massage techniques such as rubbing and applying pressure also prevent the pain sensation from reaching the receptors in the brain. An example of this response is the reduction in the degree of pain that results from rubbing an area that has been struck.

Stress

When a person experiences significant stress in his or her life, it causes physiological and psychological changes in the body. At the physiological level, heart rates can increase, adrenaline rises, sweating may occur, and tightness can be felt within the muscles of the body as the skin prepares for a "fight or flight" response. Psychologically, a person may feel overwhelmed, depressed, moody, or sad, and may even take drastic measures to deal with the stress, such as consuming alcohol or using drugs. Massage is indicated as a means to help alleviate negative stress through the personal human contact inherent in treatment, and through ridding the body of toxins and waste in the cells. During the initial massage therapy consultation, the practitioner should be aware of any indicators of extreme stress and outline a plan that will bring relaxation to the client in a timely manner. At no point should the practitioner assume the role of a psychotherapist or counselor.

Differentiation between pain and stress

Pain causes sensations that range from slight to severe. It indicates potential damage to the tissues or possible destruction within the body. Pain can be an indication of damage to nerve endings that lie beneath the surface of the skin, damage to the periosteum of the bones, damage to blood vessels and arteries, and finally, deeper damage to internal organs and muscles. The body's response to pain is both physical and physiological, which means that the body's response to pain mimics the reaction that the body has to stress. Stress is any condition that causes strain on the body or tension within the body. It can affect the internal balance and harmony within the body. Stress affects each person differently at varying levels. Overall, increased stress can be detrimental to the health of the individual. The body's reactions to stress include an increased heart rate, the secretion of "flight or flight" hormones from the adrenal gland, deeper breathing, and increased blood pressure.

Dopamine and serotonin

During a massage, some of the chemicals released within the body produce positive physiological effects. Neurotransmitters such as dopamine and serotonin are released, which contribute to pain control and mood elevation. One neurotransmitter is dopamine, which helps to control the brain's emotions, motor skills, and feelings of pleasure or pain. Serotonin is another type of neurotransmitter that also helps regulate moods, behavior, appetite, and memory. Low levels of serotonin can contribute to depression, anxiety, sleep disorders, and even personality disorders. Massage helps to increase the levels of these neurotransmitters within the body and leads to a sense of peacefulness and calmness that can help reduce stress. Massage also contributes to appetite control and increased functioning of the immune system.

Therapeutic massage and anatomy and physiology

Therapeutic massage is defined as the process of applying techniques such as effleurage, pétrissage, stretching, and stroking on the muscular structure of the body to ease pains in the tendons, ligaments, muscles, and surface of the skin. This type of massage is intended to create a sense of calmness and relaxation, as well as to alleviate any pain, stiffness, or soreness in the body. Increased circulation, greater flexibility, improved muscle tone, and improved posture are additional effects that therapeutic massage has on the body. Having a basic understanding of human anatomy allows the massage therapist to focus on the parts of the body that require additional consideration and enables him to avoid measures that can cause pain to the client. Physiological changes include the lowering of the client's blood pressure, reduction in the heart rate, and slower, deeper breathing, all of which contribute to the relaxed state of the client.

Massage movements

The basic massage movements are as follows:
- Touch – includes superficial and deep massage
- Gliding or effleurage movements – moving the hand or forearm over the body while applying varying amounts of pressure; can be aura stroking, superficial, or deep
- Kneading – includes pétrissage, rolling, lifting, and squeezing of the skin
- Friction – causing one layer of skin tissue to rub against another; can be performed by rolling, compressing, wringing, and vibrating
- Percussion – alternately striking the surface of the skin through cupping, slapping, tapping, and beating
- Joint movements – manipulating the limbs of the body through passive or active movements

Touch

Touch is defined as the action of initiating skin-to-skin contact between the massage therapist's hand and the client's body. Touch does not involve any movement. The pressure can range from extremely light to deep pressure, depending on the type of reaction the therapist is trying to achieve. Touch can have a calming physiological effect on the client. The massage therapist should open the massage session with a few moments of touch as a means of connecting with the client and becoming comfortable with his personal body space. This gentle touching is also performed at the end of the massage to signal the end of the session and provide a sense of closure for both the client and the therapist. Deep pressure can also be applied through touch. In this sense, touch is applied to calm, anesthetize, or stimulate the muscles. It is often used to soothe muscle spasms or alleviate pain. Force is applied through body movements rather than by relying only upon the strength of the therapist's arms.

Techniques

Gliding Techniques

Ethereal stroking and feather stroking
The types of movements that are based on maneuvering the hand over the client's body with varying degrees of pressure are known as gliding techniques. Ethereal or aura stroking is the process in which the practitioner glides his hands over the length of the client's body, but does not actually touch the body. The intention of this practice, according to some philosophies, is to smooth over the energy field that surrounds the body. A second type of gliding technique is feather stroking, which involves making long, gentle strokes from the center of the body outward.

Effleurage and deep gliding
Effleurage is a common Swedish massage technique that calls for successive strokes over a long surface of the body. The pressure is increased with each stroke. Superficial gliding involves applying light pressure to the body with the hand over all surfaces. This gives the therapist a chance to assess the condition of the muscles prior to commencing the massage. The amount of pressure exerted, the part of the hand that is used, and the way that the pressure is applied must all be considered when the deep gliding technique is being performed. Deep gliding strokes are designed to stretch and broaden the muscle tissue and fascia. It is best to make these movements towards the heart to encourage blood and lymph flow.

Pétrissage

Kneading, or pétrissage, is used on the fleshy parts of the body to bring about movement of fluid in deep tissues and help stretch the muscle tissue. The skin is generally raised between the hands and kneaded with firm pressure in circular motions. Often, both hands are used to perform this motion. In the type of pétrissage known as fulling, the tissue is lifted up and then spread out to enhance the area in between the muscular tissue. Another form of pétrissage is called skin rolling. In this method, the fingers pick up the skin in alternate motions and gently pull it away from the underlying tissues to create a stretching of the fascia. This motion warms the skin and helps to remove any buildup of adhesions on the tissue.

Circular and cross-fiber friction

Friction helps to move the superficial layers of tissue against the deeper tissues within the body. The action of applying friction creates warmth when the therapist presses tissue upon tissue, thereby flattening it, releasing fluids from the tissue, and also stretching it at the same time. The warmth produced also causes the client's metabolic rate to increase. Types of friction methods include circular friction and cross-fiber friction. As the name implies, circular friction involves moving the fingers or hands over the client's skin in a circular pattern. Cross-fiber friction is performed in a sharp, transverse direction to the muscle being worked on. This is the preferred method used when a specific muscle group is being rehabilitated; it promotes the rebuilding of elastic tissue fibers.

Percussion techniques

Slapping and tapping
Percussion movements are quick, striking motions that are made alternately against the body. This technique serves to stimulate the body. The movements do not involve the application of great force. The types of percussion movements are slapping, tapping, cupping, hacking, and beating. Slapping involves applying pressure from the flat palm of the hand against the surface of the body. Tapping involves using the fingertips in such a way that only the pads of the fingers come in contact with the body. The fingers can be either held in a flexed position or straight. Either way, the pressure applied is very light.

<u>Cupping, hacking, and beating</u>
Cupping involves shaping the hand into a curved shape prior to applying it to the body. This method is generally used on the rib area, and is a technique commonly used by respiratory therapists to eliminate build up and congestion in the lungs. Hacking is the use of the ulnar side of the hands to strike the body, which causes an improvement in circulation and relaxation. Beating involves using loose fists to gently pound the body, and is considered the heaviest and deepest form of percussion. This technique is used primarily on the dense muscle tissues.

PJM

One type of joint movement is known as passive joint movement (PJM). It is generally performed when the client is in a relaxed state and the therapist is able to maneuver, exercise, and stretch a part of the body. PJM is also used to determine the extent of any injuries to the client and to determine the exact range of motion that part of the body can achieve. Working the muscle and joint in this way allows the therapist to help improve the mobility of the joint and extend its range of motion. To perform the passive joint movement, the therapist must take care to move the limb only in the direction that it is designed to move, without any forceful or sharp gestures. If the movement is being done to assess damage, stopping at the point of the client's pain is indicated. To rehabilitate the joint, further extension of the limb is recommended.

AJM

In active joint movement (AJM), the client is responsible for contracting the muscle to perform the required movement of the joint. It is commonly used as an assessment tool to determine the exact capabilities and the range of motion of the client. The results can be benchmarked at the start of treatment, with a comparison made at the end of treatment to note the progress made. Active assistive joint movement is performed when the client attempts to move the joint through a series of movements. The therapist assists when the client no longer has the strength or ability to move the injured limb further. This is primarily a therapeutic device designed to restore mobility in the limb. Another type of joint movement is active resistive joint movement. In this action, the therapist or practitioner applies resistive force against the motion of the limb. This allows for the buildup of muscle strength that, in turn, leads to increased use of the limb. Resistive motions such as these can be applied to any body part.

Heat applications

Massage therapists use a number of heat applications to stimulate circulation and alleviate tissue soreness. For the most part, heat applications involve moist heat in the form of hot baths and hot towels. At all times, a massage therapist needs to be careful not to burn the client or raise the body temperature excessively. These days, massage therapists typically use silica gel packs, which can be reused between clients. Hot applications should never be placed under the body and should not cover more than 1/5 of the surface area of the body so that they do not affect body temperature. In general, hot applications are best used on specific, localized areas, such as when a client is experiencing tension or stiffness in a particular part of the body.

Cold applications

Massage therapists use cold applications to reduce body temperature, diminish circulation, and numb a particular area of the body. Cold applications may take the form of compresses (cold, wet cloths) or direct applications of ice. Applying ice to a particular part of the body for 10 minutes can reduce a client's sensitivity to pain a great deal. Ice also diminishes inflammation. Inflammation should only be treated with the ice when the massage therapist is certain of its origin. At no time should more than 1/5 of the client's body be subjected to a cold application, as this can dangerously affect body temperature. When the cold application is being used, the massage therapist should remove it every two or three minutes to make sure the skin is not blistering.

Important terms

- Compression is the rhythmic movement of the hands or fingers on the muscular tissue. Palmar compression is directed onto the muscles transverse from the bone. It does not require the use of oils or lotions and, in fact, can be performed over clothing. It is commonly used in sports massage.
- Rolling is the method in which a body part is rapidly passed back and forth between the hands. This results in warmth and encourages relaxation of the deeper muscle tissue.
- Chucking is the process by which the tissue is grabbed between the hands and moved up and down along the length of the bone. This method is performed rather quickly.
- Wringing is a process that is similar to wringing water from a towel. The hands move in opposing directions as the flesh is twisted against the bone.
- Vibration is a movement that is performed either manually or in conjunction with a device that produces continuous trembling movements against the muscle. This action helps to desensitize and numb the area.
- End feel – This occurs when the practitioner moves a client's joint through the range of motion and, just before the end point, feels a change in the quality of the movement. This sense of resistance, whether attributable to physiologic or anatomic factors, is known as the end feel.
- Hard end feel – This is the feeling of bone rubbing against bone. A common location where this occurs is in the elbow joint.
- Soft end feel – This is the limitation that occurs when moving a joint due to the location of soft tissue, which prevents additional movement.
- Empty end feel – This is the presence of pain when moving a joint, which ends up causing restrictions on the full range of motion.

Client Assessment and Treatment Planning

Consultation

Although the most important consultation will occur at the beginning of the therapeutic relationship, a massage therapist still needs to include some consultation in every meeting with a client. To begin with, the therapist needs to find out how the self-care regimen is going. If there has been any change in the client's medical status, the therapist needs to be informed of this at the beginning of the session. Also, the therapist should solicit feedback about the last session. It is always a good idea to review the short-term and long-term goals of treatment and to ensure that the client is confident and optimistic about reaching these goals. Finally, every massage session should include an opportunity for the client to bring up any issues he or she feels are relevant to treatment.

Intake forms

Most massage therapists have their clients fill out what is called an intake form during the first appointment; the completed form contains the client's entire medical history. The form includes information about past problems, current health information, and a history of illness, injury, and medical procedures. Many massage therapists include an informed consent section as part of the intake form. If the client is on any medication, this should be indicated on the intake form. The intake form is also a good place to record the client's basic personal identification information, including their name, date of birth, address, and telephone number. It is a good idea to store intake forms in an accessible location so that they can be updated in the future.

SOAP form

Most massage therapists use what is called a SOAP form to record information about individual massage sessions. The name is an acronym for the four sections of the form: Subjective, Objective, Activity, and Plan. In the subjective section, the massage therapist lists the description given by the client. In the objective section, the massage therapist lists all of his or her important observations, including the results of the postural assessment, range of motion assessment, and gait assessment. In the activity section, the massage therapist describes the procedures that were performed during the session. In the plan section, the massage therapist indicates the future activities that should be performed in subsequent sessions.

Anterior postural assessment

A comprehensive postural assessment begins with an anterior postural assessment, in which the massage therapist looks at the front of the client's body. The assessment is performed by evaluating a series of physical landmarks. First, a massage therapist will note whether the ears are at the same level; then, he or she will check to see if the nose and chin lie on the midsagittal line. The massage therapist will then check to see if the clavicles are even, and whether the sternum and belly button fall on the midsagittal line. The therapist then checks to see if the hands, which are dropped by the client's side, are at the same level, and whether the arches of the feet are roughly symmetrical. Any deviations should be noted on the postural assessment form.

Posterior postural assessment

After assessing a client's anterior posture, the massage therapist will need to assess the posterior and lateral postures. A posterior assessment begins in the same manner as the anterior assessment: checking to see if the client's ears are level. The therapist will then check to see if the client's shoulders form a line that is parallel to the ground, and whether the spine appears to run along the midsagittal line. As with the anterior assessment, the next step of the posterior assessment is to determine whether the client's pelvis is level, and whether his or her hands dangle to the same height. Finally, the therapist will assess the client's legs to determine whether the musculature is flexed in a symmetrical manner and whether the client's weight seems to be evenly distributed between his or her feet.

Lateral postural assessment

After completing the anterior and posterior postural assessments, the massage therapist will need to perform the lateral postural assessment. This begins by determining whether the client's head is properly positioned. The ears should be slightly behind the vertical reference line, which runs just in front of the lateral malleolus. The client's shoulders should be centered directly on the vertical reference line, and his or her hands should naturally face in the medial direction. Finally, the client's knees should be positioned so that the middle of the joint is on the vertical reference line. In general, the lateral postural assessment confirms problems with posture that were noted during the anterior and posterior assessments. The most common problem noted during a lateral postural assessment is that the head and neck are bent too far forward.

Gait assessment

Typically, a massage therapist will follow up the postural assessment with a brief gait assessment (walking assessment). The client will be directed to slowly walk in a straight line. The massage therapist will need to observe the client from the front, back, and side in order to collect the proper information. The client should be instructed to walk as naturally as possible. The therapist will be looking for even, symmetrical steps. The weight should be directed away from the arches of the feet. The therapist will also be looking to see if the client's head is positioned properly (above the spine), and if the shoulders are held back. The arms should swing away from the body at the exact same length and speed, and each knee should bend the same amount during a step.

Palpation assessment

During an introductory assessment of a new client, the massage therapist will need to use palpation to determine the client's problems and needs. Palpation is the use of touch to identify the structural characteristics of an individual's body. When a massage therapist performs a palpation assessment, he or she is primarily focusing on four elements: temperature, texture, movement, and rhythm. It's important to use light touch while performing a palpation assessment. Also, any palpation done on one side of the body should also be done on the other side. Palpation may be either superficial or, if necessary, quite deep. A deep palpation should not be performed unless it is necessary, as it may be painful for the client.

Basic range of motion assessment

The basic range of motion assessment is an essential part of the introductory massage session. There are two components of this assessment: active range of motion assessment and passive range of motion assessment. During the active range of motion assessment, the client will be flexing his or her joints without any assistance. The client should move slowly, and the only joint in motion should be the one being assessed. The client should proceed until he or she feels significant resistance, whether in the form of pain or tension. During a passive range of motion assessment, which is performed after the active range of motion assessment, the massage therapist will manipulate the joint without any assistance from the client. While manipulating the client's joints, the massage therapist should use gentle pressure and be responsive to any indications of pain or stress.

Temperature and texture of tissue

When performing a palpation assessment, the massage therapist will be sensitive to changes in temperature and tissue texture. The temperature of tissue is a good indicator of circulation. Warm tissue is receiving adequate blood flow, while tissue may be cold in areas affected by ischemia. As for texture, it is common for healthy muscles to move freely and feel firm but yielding. A tense muscle, on the other hand, will be knotty and resistant to movement. A healthy muscle will expand and yield in response to external pressure, while an unhealthy muscle will seem to melt away when force is applied. Moreover, an unhealthy muscle will be more likely to hurt when pressure is applied to it.

Movement and rhythm

A thorough palpation assessment will include tests to determine range of motion. It is typical for a massage therapist to palpate a joint as it is in motion. For example, the therapist might palpate the elbow as the arm is bending. If a muscle is resistant to movement or cannot relax enough to allow a normal range of motion, this is an indication of hypertonic muscle tissue. During the palpation assessment, the massage therapist must be aware of the client's breathing rhythm, heart rate, and craniosacral rhythm. It is better for the client's breathing to be slow and deep than shallow and fast. As a client relaxes, his or her breathing should slow down and deepen. It is also a good idea to check the heart rate at different points in the body, as restricted blood flow may be indicated by a slower pulse. The craniosacral flow is the motion of cerebrospinal fluid around the spinal cord and brain. It can be checked by palpating the occipital, parietal, and temporal bones.

Basic components of a treatment plan

After assessing the client and performing an initial treatment, the massage therapist and client will work together to develop a treatment plan. In order to be considered complete, a plan for future treatment needs to include the following information: proposed length of treatment (including frequency and duration of sessions), treatment techniques to be used, recommendations for self-care, and any supplemental care required by the patient. The treatment plan must be agreed upon by both the massage therapist and the client. Oftentimes, a massage therapist and client will develop a list of short-term and long-term goals, in part so that the client can recognize the gains that are being made through regular massage therapy.

Length of treatment
When developing a plan for future treatment, a massage therapist and his or her clients need to agree upon the appropriate duration and frequency of future sessions. In order to do this, it will be necessary to ascertain the amount of healing time the client will require between sessions. Clients who are under a great deal of stress or in bad health will require more healing time between sessions. If an individual is in good health, eats well, and has a relatively low stress lifestyle, he or she can be scheduled for more frequent and longer sessions. In the initial session, the massage therapist should be conscious of the point at which the client begins to experience pain. With this in mind, future sessions should be scheduled so that they will not run too long. Encouraging clients to maintain a healthy lifestyle outside of the massage environment will enable them to receive more treatment and better results from treatment.

Adjustments to a treatment plan

The initial plan for future treatment will probably be devised during the first or second massage therapy session, so it is natural for the plan to require adjustment as more information is acquired. Also, regular massage therapy will produce internal changes in the client, which may affect his or her requirements on the table. Over time, clients may develop affinities for particular techniques, which can be used more frequently during subsequent sessions. Finally, as clients begin to achieve their short-term and long-term goals, they may develop other reasons for wishing to continue massage therapy. It is a good idea to consult with a client regularly to ensure that the treatment plan is still appropriate and to make any necessary changes to improve individual results.

Types of Massages

Neuromuscular massage

Neuromuscular massage emphasizes pressure applied to the so-called "trigger points" on the body. Trigger points are areas where the nervous system can be stimulated through light touch. These points correspond to other areas of the body that can be healed through attention to the trigger points. Neuromuscular massage typically entails applying moderate pressure to the trigger points for prolonged periods of time. The goals of neuromuscular therapy are to reduce pain, correct problems with posture, and enhance range of motion. The term "neuromuscular" reflects the attention this technique gives to the interrelationship between the nervous and muscular systems.

Circulatory massage

Although most massage ends up improving the body's circulation, there are some modalities which have this as their central aim. The goal of circulatory massage is to improve the circulation of blood, lymphatic fluid, and waste products. Circulatory massage incorporates a variety of mechanical techniques that stimulate the flow of blood by improving the performance of arteries and veins. Also, there are a number of lymph drainage techniques that initiate the movement of lymph from the body tissues to the heart. A trained massage therapist will also be able to stimulate the evacuation of waste by applying specific types of pressure to the lower intestine.

Energy massage

Two of the most common forms of energy massage are Reiki and polarity therapy. Reiki aims to support the flow of energy throughout the body. The practice of Reiki is relatively easy to learn; very little formal training is required. Polarity therapy, meanwhile, seeks to improve health by making adjustments to the energy field that surrounds every human being. According to practitioners of polarity therapy, the natural circulation of electrical energy around the human body can be obstructed by imperfect body processes. These obstructions may be caused by poor posture, mood disorders, or muscular tension. The practitioner of polarity therapy tries to restore the electrical field around the subject so that he or she can regain normal energy flow.

Movement massage

Movement massage modalities oblige the client to take a more active role in his or her therapy. Some of the most common varieties of movement massage are Feldenkrais, Trager, and Alexander. Feldenkrais emphasizes relearning common movement patterns in such a way that they diminish the stresses placed on certain parts of the body. The Alexander technique is specifically aimed at improving posture and balance by forcing the client to become conscious of habitual movements. This method is especially popular among actors and dancers because of the control it gives the client over his or her body. The Trager system encourages clients to move their bodies as a therapist applies light pressure to certain key areas; this technique is good for relieving muscular tension.

Structural and postural integration massage

Structural and postural integration modalities emphasize the importance of developing and maintaining proper body alignment when standing and performing normal movements. Two of the most common modalities in this category are Rolfing and Hellerwork. Rolfing focuses on improving posture through a systematic reshaping of the body's myofascial structure. A certified "Rolfer" administers light pressure all over the body with his or her fingers, elbows, and knuckles. The goal is to relax the muscles until they reach their natural state of alignment. Hellerwork, meanwhile, focuses on releasing built-up tension in the connective tissues. According to this discipline, the body becomes used to destructive misalignment and requires massage to regain its natural structure.

Oriental massage

Oriental massage modalities emphasize the flow of energy through the body. According to their theories, the unrestricted flow of energy supports good health. Some of the most common modalities in this category are Acupressure and Shiatsu massage. Acupressure, as the name indicates, is a combination of acupuncture and massage. It involves the application of light pressure to the points of the body which, in acupuncture, are pierced with needles. Shiatsu is a similar therapy that involves treating the entire body. Shiatsu theory asserts that by restoring the overall health of the body, particular areas of stress and tension can be alleviated. Shiatsu involves the application of light pressure to the acupuncture sites in the hope that it will restore effective energy flow through the body.

Reflexology

Reflexology is a study that involves stimulating certain parts of the body to produce a reaction in other parts of the body. It is based on the principal that every organ within the body has a corresponding point on either the hands or feet. By applying pressure to the ball of the foot, for example, the practitioner can produce a favorable reaction within the lungs and heart. In addition to the organs, reflexology can also affect glands and muscles. Through the application of pressure to the areas corresponding to these glands, tension can be relieved, and there may be an overall increase in body function. As an example, the heel of the foot is believed to correspond to the lower back. Pressure on the big toe can lead to relief from headaches. It is important to understand that some skeptics do not believe that this type of massage is beneficial. In any case, practitioners should not project the opinion that reflexology is a medical cure-all.

Chair massage

Chair massage originated in Japan and is believed to be several centuries old. It is a form of massage that has become increasingly popular. It can be found in shopping malls, airports, workplaces, convention centers, and other areas where large numbers of people congregate. Chair massage allows the client to be fully clothed while sitting in a chair in a semi-reclined, prone position. Chair massage is an effective way to introduce massage to a person who may exhibit adverse reactions to touch, and is it also suitable for those who may consider traditional Swedish massage too invasive.

<u>Advantages of chair massage</u>
Chair massage is often an introduction to massage therapy for individuals who, for one reason or another, are apprehensive about the process. Chair massage is sometimes used as a way to introduce positive reactions to touch. It may be suitable for those who have been victims of sexual, physical, or emotional abuse. The chair massage technique enables the practitioner to complete a session in less than 30 minutes, thus making it readily accessible to those on a tight schedule. Finally, chair massage is more cost-effective than standard massage sessions, allowing it to be used by people who are less inclined or able to spend money on weekly massages.

<u>Procedure for performing chair massage</u>
Due to the high volume of massages being performed by chair massage practitioners, the initial consultation will likely be shorter than in a standard therapeutic setting. However, the practitioner should still screen for any contraindications to the massage prior to commencement. As the client is fully clothed and seated in a prone position, certain techniques, including effleurage and gliding, are not possible. Due to the nature of chair massage, friction, percussion, and deep touches are the only appropriate techniques. With the client seated in the prone position, the head, neck, shoulders, back, and hips may be the only areas the practitioner can access.

<u>Special considerations and hygienic practices</u>
Some chair massages require the therapist to take special considerations into account in order to provide adequate therapeutic benefits to the client. In some cases, the client is seated in a supine position to enable the therapist to gain access to the lower legs and feet to perform massage in those areas. After each client leaves, the practitioner must ensure the chair meets standards of cleanliness before the next client is seated. Wiping down areas that come into contact with the client's skin with an anti-bacterial cleanser is important to control transmission of bacteria or germs. As an alternative, disposable coverings for the face cushion can be used.

Lymph massage

Lymph massage is closely related to Swedish massage. It is designed to assist with the movement of the lymphatic fluids within the body. When lymph nodes are filled with fluid, a condition known as lymphedema, physicians sometimes recommend lymph drainage massage as a means of alleviating the symptoms. Specific methods designed to assist with the flow of lymph fluids can cause an increase in metabolism, drain stagnant fluids and toxins, and stimulate the immune system. The rhythmic movements used in lymph massage also stimulate the parasympathetic nervous system which, in turn, helps to relieve stress, depression, and insomnia. Lymph massage can also help rebalance the chemistry within the body, assist in tissue regeneration, normalize organs, and boost the immune system. When done correctly, the procedure entails gentle, slow movements that are performed over the lymph nodes in a circular pattern. Light pressure is then applied in the direction of lymph flow to direct the movement of lymph.

Deep tissue massage

Deep tissue massage targets the tissues of the body that are below the superficial musculature. Some of the most common forms of deep tissue massage include cross-fiber friction, connective tissue massage, craniosacral massage, and myofascial massage. A deep tissue massage generally includes long strokes of moderate intensity and prolonged periods of pressure to certain points on the body. In order to apply direct contact to the deep muscles of the body, a certain degree of relaxation must be achieved. Therefore, it may take a while before attention can be directed to the deep muscles. Deep tissue massage can be painful, so the client should be monitored closely during each session.

Deep tissue massage refers to the massage style that focuses on the deeper muscles and fascia tissues. Various techniques are used in this form of massage to alleviate any tension in the muscular fibers. Massage of this nature can also contribute to psychological and physiological changes in the body. These therapeutic techniques may require long warm-up periods before the deep tissues of the client can be accessed. The intent behind this type of massage is to loosen the bonds between the layers of connective tissue. Some of the popular deep massage techniques are Rolfing, Trager, Hellerwork, and Feldenkrais.

<u>Rolfing</u>
One type of deep tissue massage, known as Rolfing, is named after Dr. Ida Rolf, the woman who developed the technique. She devised this technique to alleviate tension and structural problems caused by years of poor posture and alignment. Rolfing utilizes a heavy-handed technique to realign the body. Performed over a series of many treatments, the massage therapist uses his or her hands, fists, or even knuckles to align the body's movements and create a sense of balance within. A full treatment of Rolfing involves a series of 10 treatments, although fewer treatments can also lead to improvement.

Trigger point therapy

Trigger points in the body refer to skeletal muscle areas that are hyperirritable. The presence of palpable nodules in the bands of muscle fibers sometimes causes pain responses that can refer to other parts of the body. Trigger points are classified according to their location in the body and whether or not pain is felt upon palpitation. A common trigger point site is an acupuncture site, though some trigger points are located elsewhere on the body. Activation of a trigger point can be caused by an increase in stress levels, overuse of a particular muscle, and even an arthritic condition. A brief listing of common trigger points is given below:
- Active myofascial trigger point
- Latent myofascial trigger point
- Central trigger point
- Attachment trigger point
- Primary (or key) trigger point
- Satellite trigger point
- Associate trigger point

Acupressure

Similar in theory to acupuncture, acupressure is a Chinese technique in which pressure is applied from the hand, elbow, or fingers to acupuncture points across the body. The purpose of acupressure is to relieve the body by balancing the physical and psychological aspects. Through this method, a person can experience an increase in circulatory function and an enhanced ability to manage pain. Acupressure is usually part of an overall health regimen that also incorporates a healthy diet, exercise, and meditation. The overall goal is to develop a holistic lifestyle. Areas of the body where pressure points may be found are along the crown of the head, the temple, the forehead, and the upper jaw. Other areas can include the sides and front of the neck, upper arms, elbow joint, and the outside of the thighs and lower legs. Areas that commonly experience feelings of relief through acupressure include the toes, metatarsals, ankles, heels, and Achilles tendon.

Hydrotherapy, heat therapy, and cold treatments

Hydrotherapy is the practice of using water in its liquid, gas, or solid forms as part of a massage therapy treatment plan. Heat therapy can involve the application of dry heat, moist heat, or diathermy. Dry heat involves the use of heating pads, infrared radiation, or a sauna. Moist heat can come from an immersion bath, spray, heat packs, or a steam bath. Diathermy can entail the transmission of shortwave or microwave electromagnetic fields onto the tissue. The purpose of heat therapy is to cause vessels to dilate and increase circulation. Care must be taken to closely monitor the client's body temperature. Cold therapy is also known as cryotherapy. This technique is performed to help reduce the edema, swelling, and pain accompanying an injury. Cold treatments should be applied for short periods of time due to the possibility of tissue injury from the cold. Examples of cold treatments are immersion baths, ice packs, ice massage, mechanical compressors, and vasocoolant sprays.

When used as a method of therapy, water can be used in any of its three forms: solid, liquid, or gaseous vapor. When cold water is used for hydrotherapy, it has the immediate effect of cooling the skin and drawing blood away from the surface of the body. The nerves experience a reduction in their sensitivity levels and the activity of the body's cells in that particular area begins to slow down. After these initial reactions take place, a secondary reaction occurs, which causes the skin to become warmer and more relaxed. The blood cells on the surface of the skin begin to expand again and nerve impulses increase. The activity level of nearby cells increases. When heat therapy is conducted, reactions that occur cause the blood cells from the interior of the body to move towards the surface of the skin, which produces a reddish area on the skin. These blood vessels dilate and cause an increase in circulation. The body's temperature rises, and sweating may occur. All of these changes serve to relax the blood vessels, nerves, and muscles.

57

Aromatherapy

Aromatherapy is the use of essential oils from natural herbs, flowers, and spices to enhance the massage experience through the sense of smell. These aromas can bring about a specific reaction, and are commonly chosen to augment the massage session. Some of the most popular essential oils are chamomile, eucalyptus, jasmine, lavender, and lemongrass. The effects these oils produce can be calming, stimulating, refreshing, or relaxing. It is not a good idea to use these essential oils at their full strength. Instead, they should be combined with another medium, such as carrier oil. This oil serves as a lubricant and helps to blend the oil so it is not overly concentrated, which can cause irritation. Aromatherapy can also involve the use of scented candles or lotion. Prior to the massage, the therapist should consult the intake form or ask the client verbally about any allergies or sensitivities to oils or aromas that may be used during the massage.

Body wraps

Body wraps are used for different purposes, including relaxation, detoxification, and cleansing and softening the skin. Various substances can be used in the wraps, including seaweed, volcanic clay, and mud. Heat is a common element of wraps, whether it comes from an outside source or is obtained from the body. Contraindicators for wraps include high blood pressure, heart disease, and pregnancy. Body wraps are beneficial in that they provide comfort, security, and warmth, and also allow the nutrients to be absorbed in a closed environment instead of being dispersed through the air.

Technique for performing a body wrap

When performing a body wrap, the practitioner must be aware of factors that may prevent the client from being fully wrapped. The practitioner must also take precautions when determining the temperature level of the wrap. The table is laid out with a blanket, a thermal blanket, a towel, and finally, a plastic wrap. The client lies down on this plastic and an exfoliation is performed on the client's skin prior to the application of the seaweed or mud. As the seaweed or mud is brushed over the body, the practitioner wraps that portion of the body to prevent heat from escaping. Upon completion, the client is completely engulfed in wraps and is allowed to relax for some time before being assisted through the clean-up process by the therapist.

Exfoliation procedure

An exfoliation procedure can be performed in a massage therapy room. In this instance, the body is moistened with a sponge rather than in a shower or bath. After the body has been moistened, the practitioner puts salts or exfoliates into his hands and applies them in a circular fashion over the body. Only one surface is exfoliated at a time. A wet towel is used to wipe off the salts, and then a wet loofah is used to apply soap to the body. After the body has been cleansed, another hot, wet cloth is used to remove all residue of soap. The body is then dried off with another towel, and the practitioner then applies moisturizer all over the body. Exfoliation using salts from the Dead Sea is similar in nature, except the salts are mixed with water to form a paste prior to applying them to the body.

Athletic or sports massage

Athletic massage is used to help treat athletic injuries, which increases the level of strength training, conditioning, and activity. The sports massage therapist must be knowledgeable about anatomy, physiology, kinesiology, and biomechanics in order to help the athlete return to the level of conditioning required for his sport. Biomechanics refers to the movement of the body. Soft tissue injuries commonly account for a large portion of the injuries seen by the sports massage therapist. Sports massage therapists must have knowledge of the various muscle groups and how they are used within the sport. It is also important for him to understand the functions of the circulatory system and the nervous system, as they also interact with the muscles.

<u>Beneficial effects</u>
The main effects of an athletic massage are:
- Oxygen is more readily available, which allows for repair of the injured body part.
- Waste materials are flushed out by increased circulation, causing increased energy levels.
- The muscles, ligaments, and tendons are stretched, allowing for greater flexibility.
- The occurrence of muscle spasms is reduced.
- Adhesions are broken down within the muscle, resulting in less scar tissue formation after an injury.
- Collagen fibers come into alignment, leading to a stronger healed area.
- The likelihood of future injuries is reduced.
- Acids are released from the body, which causes the muscles to "bounce" back after an intense workout.
- The career of an athlete can potentially be extended because they may sustain fewer injuries.

When performing a warm-up massage on an athlete, it is important to note any potential problems that could lead to a more serious, debilitating injury. If an injury does occur, massage can help to alleviate the common problems associated with the injury. Massage is an effective means of reducing edema and swelling of the affected joint or area. The time that the body needs to recover from the injury is minimized. The scar tissue that is formed at the site of the injury is more flexible, which means the tissue is less stiff. The athlete can develop an increased range of motion in the affected limb as a result of continued massage. The athlete stands a greater chance of returning to full form more quickly than if massage was not included as part of the rehabilitation program.

<u>Components of athletic massage</u>
An athletic massage is broken down into four parts: pre-event massage, post-event massage, restorative or training massage, and rehabilitation massage. Pre-event massage is used before a competition to prepare and invigorate the athlete for the rigors of a competition. It is usually given between 15 minutes to 4 hours before a competition to increase flexibility and circulation. A post-event massage helps to cool the body down and restore the tissues to their normal state. The kneading, compression, and light stretching also helps to relax the athlete. A restorative massage is used during training, and includes deep cross-fiber friction and joint stretches. Rehabilitation massage is used to help heal and repair muscle tissue after an injury. This type of massage shortens the recuperative time and also prevents any scar tissue from forming. It helps build a stronger muscle or joint, and also allows the athlete to return to training with less likelihood of re-injury.

Business Practices

Self-employed

One of the first decisions that must be made after being certified as a massage therapist is whether to go into business for oneself or work as an employee at a spa, doctor's office, or medical facility. There are pros and cons to each situation. Working as a self-employed massage therapist forces the practitioner to be responsible for paying his own employment taxes, paying for needed supplies (such as office equipment and the massage table), and assuming any rental costs for the facility. Disadvantages include the lack of a formal support team, being responsible for managing the paperwork for the business side as a self-employed entity, and the lack of a steady paycheck due to the time needed to build the business. Working in an established environment allows the therapist to have a built-in clientele, without incurring the overhead costs of doing business. Additionally, the therapist has the support of fellow employees to help with increased client loads. The company would also provide benefits such as vacation, sick leave, and health insurance, and would be responsible for paying any state and federal employer taxes.

Types of businesses

A massage therapist has the option of registering their business as a sole proprietor, partnership, limited liability corporation, or corporation. There are advantages and disadvantages to each of these arrangements. A sole proprietorship is a business in which the owner assumes all responsibility for the business, whether from a financial or obligatory standpoint. The individual is also legally responsible for all failures of the business and may be held accountable if any lawsuits are brought against the company. The courts will see the individual and the business as one entity. Therefore, the person is held legally responsible for any business debt. An advantage of a sole proprietorship is that the owner is not accountable to a board or group of shareholders. Under a partnership, two or more individuals share in the successes and failures of the business; all partners share equally in the risk. It is similar to a sole proprietorship in that the group of owners can be held personally responsible for all activities of the business. A limited liability corporation (LLC) is a combination of a partnership and a corporation. A limited liability corporation has some of the same benefits as a corporation, but there is less paperwork involved. Additionally, an LLC offers more protection of one's personal assets in the event of a lawsuit. Finally, a corporation assigns management of the business to a board of directors who share in the policy development and decision-making processes. Stockholders are financially tied to the success of the company, as they share in any profits that are made.

Start-up expenses

As with any business, money is needed to buy the necessary office equipment and to help cover the costs of leasing space. Start-up expenses for a massage therapy practice can include the following:
- Work location – While leasing office space is more expensive than working from one's home, safety concerns may drive many therapists to find space to share with other therapists.
- Utilities – This refers to the costs associated with electricity, water, gas, phone lines, etc. that will be required in the work space.
- Massage therapy tables and other equipment – This can include portable as well as stationary massage tables and chairs, bolsters, towels and linens, and massage oils and lotions. It can also include any hydrotherapy tubs and other equipment used to perform percussive and vibratory movements on the client.
- Furniture – Desk and chairs are needed for the waiting area, office, and conference room. The massage therapist also requires a personal work desk.
- Office supplies – Required supplies could include a computer, fax machine, file cabinets, writing utensils, appointment books, etc.
- Advertising and printing expenses – These are the costs of marketing your massage therapy business, whether through print, TV, or radio advertisements.
- Insurance and licensing costs – These help the practitioner limit liabilities and ensure they are able to remain in business.

Licenses and permits

In order to successfully operate a business, several licenses must be obtained. These include:

- Fictitious name statement (DBA) – This is required to differentiate between the owner's name and the name of the business. This form is filed with the county clerk's office to prevent other individuals from securing the exact same business name.
- Business license – This is required to operate a business within a city.
- Massage license – This allows the practitioner to receive fees for massage services.
- Sales tax permit – This is required if the practitioner sells products or charges tax on services.
- Planning and zoning permits – These are required to ensure that the business meets the zoning requirements for that area, especially if the business is run out of the owner's home.
- Building safety permit – After an inspection to determine that a facility is safe for use by both employees and clients, a building permit is issued in the name of the business.
- Employers Identification Number (EIN) – This is a number assigned to the business for federal tax purposes. This is required only by partnerships and businesses that hire employees.
- Provider's number – An ID number to help identify a specific practitioner for the purposes of insurance paperwork and claims information.

Insurance

In addition to purchasing insurance to address the risks of fire and theft, the massage therapist practitioner also needs to consider other types of insurance to protect the business.

- Liability insurance covers the business in the event of any injuries on the property, or if litigation is brought against the business. If the business is run out of the home, some of these incidents may be covered under the homeowner's policy.
- Professional liability insurance guards against the possibility of litigation being brought forth by a client who feels that the practitioner caused injury or harm because they were negligent while providing services.
- Automobile insurance covers the passengers and the vehicle in the event of an accident. Coverage ranges from liability only to full coverage, regardless of fault. This insurance should be obtained as an individual, but also if a vehicle is used for business purposes and travel.
- Worker's compensation insurance covers those employees who have been hired to work for the practitioner if they become injured while on the job.
- Medical and health insurance can also be provided for the owner/practitioner and all of his employees.
- Disability insurance covers any employees who become disabled due to injuries sustained on the job.

Business ethics

In order to run a successful and ethical massage therapy practice, the massage therapist should adhere to the following guidelines to provide the best possible level of service to his or her clientele. Presenting oneself professionally, both in attitude and in appearance, and projecting a positive demeanor is important to make your clients feel at ease. Treating each client with the same level of respect, regardless of gender or age, also shows concern for the client, as does adhering to the schedule in order to provide ample time for each client. Additionally, being able to run one's business in an organized manner shows good business skills and allows the therapist to be attentive to the needs of their clients. Joining a professional organization shows the practitioner ways to increase his skills in the field, and also provides an opportunity for networking and professional growth. Finally, to perform in an ethical manner, the massage therapist should obey all the laws and legal requirements while doing business and keep his or her personal life separate from business affairs.

Marketing plan

Marketing is the process of promoting one's business with the intention of increasing income and building up the client base. Marketing generally takes the form of advertising, including written brochures, print ads in newspapers, websites, and other publications, and media ads featured on radio and television. Marketing can also take the form of referrals from repeat customers. A successful marketing plan focuses on the needs of the client and addresses how one's business can meet those needs. Marketing should be an on-going process, with adjustments made as some strategies are discovered to bring about more clientele than others. The types of marketing conducted are determined by the budget, time constraints, and also the time required for implementation. A marketing plan is an outline used by a business to determine the actions necessary to achieve a certain goal. Most marketing plans are created for a period of one to five years.

Employees

As the massage therapy practice grows, it may become necessary to add to one's staff to serve more clients. Some businesses hire massage therapists as independent contractors, while others hire them as full-time employees. As an independent contractor, the practitioner is responsible for paying his own taxes, and will need to file tax forms 1099 and 1096 if he exceeds $600.00 in income during the previous year. As a full-time employee, the employer is responsible for providing an hourly paycheck and a benefits package. In either case, the person hired can help the business succeed or fail, depending on his professionalism and how personable he or she is with clients. When seeking out new employees, it is important to verify all credentials and licensing, ensure that appropriate training is provided, and work with the person to help him achieve the business's goals.

Safety Practices

Appropriate hygiene regimen

In order to prevent infection and the spread of disease, a massage therapist needs to engage in a comprehensive hygiene regimen. The most important part of this regimen is handwashing after every client encounter. During handwashing, an antibacterial soap should be used. All jewelry should be removed from the hands. Alcohol-based hand sanitizers are an acceptable alternative. A therapist should also put on latex gloves whenever he or she is required to clean up the bodily fluids of a client. A therapist should clean his or her equipment regularly with antiseptics, and should occasionally use a stronger disinfectant, making sure to rinse the equipment thoroughly with warm water afterwards.

Contamination

Massage therapy can be a breeding ground for infection if the massage therapist is not careful. To maintain their clientele, a therapist must have a facility that is clean and sterile, and must protect against the spread of disease to safeguard the well-being of their clients. Following strict laws regulating sanitation procedures, the massage therapist must utilize disinfectants, antiseptics, and other cleaning agents to maintain a healthy environment. Illness- and disease-causing pathogens are transmitted from one infected person to another directly or indirectly. They can enter the body through inhalation, ingestion, broken skin, contact with mucous membranes, or sexual contact.

Transmittal of pathogens

Pathogens can be transmitted through beverages or food. Types of pathogens the massage therapist should be concerned about are bacteria, fungus, and viruses. Bacteria are most commonly found on dirty surfaces and in unclean water, and can cause illnesses such as pneumonia, typhoid fever, TB, diphtheria, and syphilis, just to name a few. Viruses can invade living hosts and transmit diseases such as colds, mumps, measles, and pneumonia. Warm, moist environments create an ideal environment for fungi and mold to reproduce. Fungal infections are responsible for ringworm, athlete's foot, and Candida.

Universal precautions

The following steps are considered necessary precautions to stop the spread of infection:
- Washing hands with soap and water before and after contact with each client
- Using disposable paper towels rather than cloth
- Washing skin and hands thoroughly if any contact is made with contaminated fluids
- Wearing gloves when performing certain tasks and washing hands after removing the gloves
- Washing any linens contaminated with blood or bodily fluids in hot water with bleach and drying them in a hot dryer
- Handling contaminated linens as little as possible and separating them from other linens
- Cleaning surfaces such as walls and ceilings with disinfectant if they come in contact with spills requiring sanitation

Maintenance of safe facilities

When we think of safety in the context of massage therapy, we usually think of the physical manipulations, which have the potential to stress and strain the body of the client or the therapist. However, it is equally important for the facilities at the massage therapist's office to be safe. By facilities, we mean all of the buildings, furnishings, and equipment used by the massage therapist and his or her customers. In order to maintain a high level of safety, a massage therapist needs to keep the buildings clean, uncluttered, well-lit, and sanitized. All equipment should be checked frequently to make sure it is sturdy and safe for use. Every massage office should have an accessible first-aid kit and the phone numbers for emergency services posted next to the telephone.

Maintaining client safety

The best way to maintain client safety is to have clean and safe facilities, and to communicate any potential hazards to the client. For instance, clients should be alerted whenever the therapist is about to position his or her body in a potentially stressful manner. Disabled or elderly clients should be assisted into position and should also be helped on and off the massage table. Clients who are ill, injured, or have severe allergies should have these conditions thoroughly examined before undergoing massage therapy. In addition, a massage therapist needs to keep a fully-stocked first-aid kit on hand at all times in case the client should suffer some injury. In order to minimize the risk of infection, the massage therapist should wash his or her hands after every client.

Maintaining therapist safety

Although a massage therapist primarily focuses on improving the quality of life of his or her clients, the therapist also needs to protect him or herself from injury or illness. To this end, the therapist should wash his or her hands after every encounter with a client. The therapist should not perform any therapies that are outside his or her scope of expertise, and should be aware of any counterindications for massage practice. In order to reduce the risk of infection in the massage environment, the therapist should clean and sterilize equipment with a disinfectant regularly. The therapist should also ensure that his or her work environment has adequate ventilation.

Physical health of massage therapist

A person considering massage therapy should understand that this profession requires a great deal of physical strength. To assist others through massage, the therapist places considerable stress on his own body, which can be injured if proper procedures are not followed when performing the massage on a client. Proper stances, exercises for the hands, and good body mechanics will help eliminate some of the stress on the practitioner. It is important to develop good posture, coordination, balance, and stamina to provide the best possible massages for the client with minimal damage to oneself. As the hands are the most important of the practitioner's tools, flexibility is key to controlling the speed of the massage and pressure sensitivity, along with the ability to conform to the contours of the client's body. Along with proper physical conditioning, the therapist should also concentrate on his emotional state during the massage and not let outside influences mar the session.

Body mechanics

In order to avoid injury and unnecessary strain on the body, a massage therapist needs to learn proper body mechanics. One of the main principles of body mechanics as it applies to massage therapy is leverage, the technique of producing the greatest amount of pressure on the client with the least amount of work. Basically, leverage is achieved in massage therapy by locking the arms at the elbows and leaning on the client so that the weight of the therapist is doing most of the work. Also, massage therapists should try to stand as close to their clients as possible, as proximity makes the work of creating pressure easier. In order to deliver effective force with the use of leverage, it is important for the massage table to be set low enough that the therapist can lean into the patient without his or her arm being at too much of an angle with his or her torso.

Symmetric and asymmetric stance

In order to avoid being injured as a result of the repetitive stresses associated with practicing massage therapy, one needs to learn the appropriate uses of the symmetric and asymmetric stances. In the symmetric stance, the feet are shoulder-width apart, with the knees flexed to the same degree and the toes pointed forward. This stance is appropriate when the client is directly in front of the therapist, as the weight is evenly distributed between the legs. In the asymmetric stance, on the other hand, one foot is in front of the other, with the front foot pointed forward and the back foot pointed slightly to the outside. In this pose, the majority of the weight is on the back foot. This stance is appropriate when the therapist is trying to get extra leverage to apply more pressure to the client's body. A massage therapist needs to be able to work comfortably with either the right or left foot forward in the asymmetric stance.

Poor body mechanics

Although massage therapy is primarily a gentle discipline, the repetitive movements and application of pressure can result in injury for therapists with poor body mechanics. In particular, the hands, wrists, and elbows are subject to a great deal of strain during massage. In order to avoid repetitive stress injuries, a therapist should keep the table at the appropriate height (such that the arms are almost fully extended when laid on the client) and avoid applying pressure with too great of an angle from the body. The therapist's back should be kept straight as much as possible, and his or her shoulders should remain back rather than hunched forward. Therapists should also slightly flex their knees and wear shoes that distribute their weight evenly throughout the foot.

Draping

Purpose

In order to preserve a client's privacy during massage, a massage therapist will drape the client's body with linens. Besides preventing embarrassment on the part of the client, draping also keeps the client warm, which improves the efficacy of massage. When performing a full body massage, the massage therapist will have to uncover and recover body parts in order to gain access to all the necessary areas. Although the precise requirements for draping vary from state to state, as a general rule, the breasts, genitals, and gluteal cleft should remain covered at all times. The most common form of draping is known as two-sheet draping; it requires one sheet to cover the massage table and another to cover the client. Some more advanced forms of draping may require additional, smaller sheets.

Top cover method

One of the more common styles of draping is known as top cover (or two-sheet) draping. It requires the use of two large sheets: one to cover the massage table and one large enough to cover the entire client. A set of quality twin bed sheets would be suitable. In a pinch, you can use a couple of large bath towels in place of the top sheet. The patient can be wrapped in the top sheet on the way from the dressing room to the massage table. One of the benefits of a large top sheet is that you can easily lift it up to block your own view, which will allow the client to maneuver into position for the next part of the massage.

Basic techniques
At the beginning of the massage, the top cover should be positioned long-ways so that only the client's head is exposed. To massage the torso of a male, simply fold the top cover down to the waist. To massage the arms, simply fold the top cover under the client's arms at the armpits. To massage the torso of a woman, place a towel or pillowcase over the breasts and slide the cover out from under it. To massage a leg, simply slide the top cover back so that only that leg is exposed. When it is time for the client to roll over, you can either hold the cover up to block your view or hold the cover in place while the client rolls beneath it.

Full-sheet method
Some massage therapists employ the full-sheet method of draping, in which only one large sheet is used to cover both the massage table and the client. A queen-size bed sheet is usually sufficient for this kind of draping. The sheet is placed on the massage table and then folded over the client. It will be necessary to give the client a separate wrap to wear from the dressing room to the massage table. Once the client has been positioned inside the full sheet, the wrap can be removed. Some massage therapists will then take the wrap and lay it across the client's chest in order to hold the full sheet in place.

Basic techniques in full-sheet
When a client has been draped according to the full-sheet method of draping, his or her arms can be massaged by discreetly sliding them out from under the top of the sheet. When they are not exposed, the client's arms should be placed at his or her sides underneath the sheet. The legs should be undraped from the foot upwards. Otherwise, the drapes on each leg should be tucked under the legs to prevent the drape from sliding off. To massage the torso of a male, fold the top cover down to the uppermost part of the pubic bone. To massage the torso of a female, place the wrap on top of the breasts and slide the top cover out from under it while the client holds the wrap in place. When the client needs to roll over, only cover him or her from the neck to the knees and hold the cover in place during the operation.

Communication during draping

The art of draping a client during massage is somewhat complex and may make a shy client uneasy. In order to reduce client anxiety, it is a good idea to maintain appropriate communication regarding the purpose of your draping movements. You should explain the intention of draping to every new client before beginning the massage. Before uncovering any part of the client's body, describe what you are about to do. Sometimes, you will need to hold up the sheet to block your own view as the client gets into a different position. You should always remind the client that you will not be able to see them and then describe the position you would like them to assume. Always give the client an opportunity to ask questions.

Office and equipment

Typical set-up

Depending on the extent of the practice and the funds available, the therapist should have basic equipment for the following areas of the practice: the office area, the massage area, and the restroom facility or hydrotherapy area. An independent massage therapist with a smaller practice will generally work out of their home or a small office. The business area should be cordoned off from clients for confidentiality purposes and to allow for privacy during client consultations. The restroom facility provides a place for clients to shower before and after the massage, and is also a place for the massage therapist to wash his or her hands between each massage. Finally, the massage area is made up of the massage table; a stool; a storage area for linens, oils, creams, etc.; and a dressing area for the client. Pillows or bolsters should be readily available to help make the client more comfortable during the massage. Appropriate drapes should be located nearby to give clients privacy during the massage.

Size, temperature, and furnishings

A typical massage room should be no less than 10 feet wide by 12 feet long in order to accommodate the massage table, desk, and storage areas for linens and lotions, and to provide enough space for the therapist to adequately maneuver around the table to perform the massage. Considering that the client will not have clothes on during the massage, it is important to keep the room at an ideal temperature to prevent chills. A temperature of 72° Fahrenheit would ensure the comfort of the client as well as the therapist, who may become overheated while performing the massage.

Ventilation, lighting, and music

In order to help their clients relax, massage therapists need to make some environmental adjustments to the massage room. Proper ventilation should be in place to provide fresh air that is free from odors. The lighting in the room should not be harsh and glaring; it should be reflective or soft, which will make the client feel comfortable. Purchasing dimmer switches to adjust lighting according to the client's needs and preferences would be a simple and worthwhile investment. Music also helps to promote relaxation; however, it is best to make music selections based on the client's preferences rather than the therapist's.

Massage table

Next to the massage therapist's hands, a massage table is one of the most important pieces of equipment. It should be determined whether the table will be used in a home setting or in an office environment. The table should be firm, stable, and comfortable for the client. A table that is an appropriate height is one that enables the therapist to place his hands flat on the surface while keeping his arms straight. This is the best height to provide leverage and help prevent fatigue of the back, neck, shoulders, and arms while performing the massage.

Many tables are made with hydraulic or manual height adjustments, which are especially useful if different therapists will be using the same table. The standard size of a massage table is approximately 29 inches wide by 68 to 72 inches long. This can accommodate most average-sized clients, but may be too short for taller individuals. The table's padding should consist of at least one to two inches of high-density foam for optimal comfort for the client. A vinyl covering is preferred over any other type of covering, due to ease of cleaning and sanitizing between clients. To care for vinyl, a solution of mild detergent is all that is needed. Some massage tables are also adjustable to accommodate patients with different needs.

Accountability

Accountability

A massage therapist must demonstrate accountability, the ability to take on the responsibilities of a professional. Being accountable means taking responsibility when massage therapy produces an adverse reaction, as well as taking credit for the positive consequences of therapy. In order to be truly accountable, one needs to fully understand the scope of the practice of massage therapy, as well as the code of ethics that must be followed by professionals. Only by understanding the rules of professional practice and the limitations on a massage therapist can one truly take responsibility and be accountable.

Ethical issue

Sooner or later, you will be required to resolve an ethical issue in your professional practice. This issue may or may not have arisen because of your own conduct. Nevertheless, it is your responsibility as an ethical professional to do everything within your power to resolve the issue. First, you should gather as much information as you need to make an informed decision. You should then determine who will be affected by your decision. If necessary, you should contact relevant law enforcement authorities. You may also find it helpful to consult the code of ethics for your jurisdiction. Finally, you should make what you consider to be the ethical decision, and then explain your decision and its consequences to all relevant parties.

Personal boundaries

Boundaries are defined as the personal comfort zones that each person maintains for his own security. Boundaries are intangible and unseen. The acceptable distance from one person's body to another individual varies and is dependent on each individual's personal preferences. Boundaries can be divided into four types: physical, emotional, intellectual, and sexual. They serve as a personal protective device and during the course of the massage the practitioner should be aware of any subtle nuances that would let him know that the client may be on the verge of discomfort. It is important that the practitioner be aware of the client's boundaries, and it is vital that they exhibit the utmost respect, concern, and professionalism at all times.

Professional boundaries

There are eight issues related to professional boundaries. They include:
- Location of services received – This refers to the location at which massage services are received. Boundaries are less likely to be crossed when the client's safety, comfort, and security are taken into consideration.
- Interpersonal space – This refers to the distance between the practitioner and the client. For sensitive individuals, it is one of the boundaries crossed most frequently.
- Appearance – The impression the massage therapist practitioner makes on their clients is influenced by their appearance. Good hygiene and modest clothing promote a sense of professionalism.
- Self-disclosure – Any personal information provided by the client to the practitioner should be directly related to the treatment and therapy at hand.

Language, touch, time, and money

There are eight issues related to professional boundaries. They include:
- Language- The choice of words, tone, phrasing, and intonation help to create a safe, secure, peaceful environment.
- Touch – Touch during a massage is necessary. However, skin-to-skin contact should only occur at the parts of the body that are being massaged. The genital area is to be avoided, and draping should be provided for all areas not being massaged.
- Time – Adherence to set appointment times shows respect for the client's time and other personal activities. Also, open communication regarding policies for missed appointments, no shows, and lateness helps to define the boundaries between the client and the practitioner.
- Money – Defining the fee schedule for services rendered in advance of the therapeutic sessions helps to define boundaries. Charging various fees based on a person's skin color, gender, relationship status, etc. does not reflect the type of professionalism all healthcare professionals should be trying to achieve.

Code of ethics

A code of ethics defines the roles and responsibilities assigned to the members of a given profession. Many of the professional organizations for massage therapists have issued codes of ethics. These codes are all somewhat different, but contain a few common elements. Massage therapists are required to strive to provide the best service to their clients, but to never administer treatment for which they have not been trained. Massage therapists are forbidden from practicing any form of discrimination when they deal with clients. They are required to obey all of the laws in their jurisdiction and to accept responsibility for their actions. They are required to act professionally at all times and to avoid conflicts of interest and unprofessional relationships with clients.

Therapeutic relationship

The relationship between a massage therapist and his or her clients is often described as a therapeutic relationship: one in which one person is responsible for improving the health and quality of life of another person in exchange for money. There is a subtle dynamic at work in this relationship, however, and therapists need to be aware of this. For one thing, it is essential to note that the client is in a significantly weaker position in the relationship. He or she is unlikely to know much about the treatment, will be placed in various compromising positions throughout the therapy, and will have to rely on the professionalism and efficacy of the therapist. The therapist should be conscious of the fact that the client has placed him or herself in a vulnerable position voluntarily and should make sure that the client's trust has been well placed. The therapist is responsible for upholding the highest professional standards and not taking advantage of the power he or she holds over the client.

Dual relationships

Occasionally, you may be required to manage a dual relationship in your professional practice. In other words, you may be required to provide professional services for a person with whom you already have a personal relationship. This is not necessarily an ethical quandary, so long as both parties are aware of the restrictions on the relationship during professional service. So long as you perform your duties as a professional according to the standards set by your employer and the relevant professional associations, it should not matter whether you are providing therapy to a friend or relative. However, you should be sure to treat your friends and family as you would any other valued client. You should also be sure that they in turn treat you with the respect you are owed as a professional.

Sexuality issues

Massage is a sensual activity, and so a massage therapist needs to be careful to maintain appropriate sexual boundaries during his or her professional work. At no time should a massage therapist come into direct contact with the genitalia of their clients. It is not uncommon for a client to become sexually aroused during the course of a massage. This is only natural, as massage tends to stimulate the parasympathetic nervous system and direct more blood flow to the genitals. One way to deal with this problem is to deliver more rapid, drumming strokes to the body, which tends to stifle arousal. Another strategy is to simply explain to the client the physiological reasons for his or her arousal and leave it at that. It is not considered sexual harassment to simply describe to a client the natural changes that occur during massage, so long as no effort is made to violate the boundary between client and therapist.

Educational requirements for certification

There are no mandated national educational requirements for certification or licensure as a massage therapist. However, there are certain elements required for certification that are common among all jurisdictions. For instance, almost all states require applicants to have a high school diploma or GED. Most licensing organizations require at least 500 hours of instruction in massage therapy, with emphasis on anatomy, physiology, pathology, modalities of bodywork and massage, contraindications for massage, massage safety, and professional practice. Usually, individuals are required to pass a standardized test in order to receive their license. There are a few different standardized tests used throughout the United States for this purpose.

Revocation or suspension of license

If you violate the code of ethics or regulations set by the governing body, you may have your massage therapist's license revoked or suspended. For instance, if you are convicted of a felony while practicing as a massage therapist, your license may be suspended. The following events can also be cause for the revocation or suspension of a license: prostitution, willful negligence, substance abuse, deceptive advertising, and sexual misconduct in the line of duty. Furthermore, if the organization that issued your license determines that you used deception in order to obtain a license, it may be revoked.

Scope of practice

A scope of practice is the list of activities a given professional has the right to perform under on his or her license. The precise description of a massage therapist's scope of practice is different in every state. It is important for a therapist to understand his or her scope of practice so that he or she does not overstep professional boundaries. The scope of practice for wellness massage is smaller than that for therapeutic massage. This is because the goals of wellness massage are more general and less ambitious. In order to practice wellness massage, a massage therapist must have general training in the anatomy, physiology, pathology, and modalities of wellness massage. He or she is then authorized to use these modalities to promote circulation and reduce stress.

Informed consent forms

Since the massage therapist understands his or her professional business much better than his or her clients, it is the responsibility of the therapist to describe in detail any proposed treatment before initiation. This is done by means of an informed consent form, in which the proposed treatment is described in full, including any potential risks of the treatment. The presentation of an informed consent document gives the client a chance to ask questions. An informed consent form may also include a list of actions which would result in the immediate termination of treatment; it is a good idea for the therapist to publish such a list in the event that a dispute with the client arises.

Professional communication skills

One of the most important but least talked about aspects of ethical professional practice as a massage therapist is effective communication. In order to serve a client, the therapist needs to be able to describe his or her work and understand the concerns, complaints, and questions of the client. The therapist needs to establish a relationship with the client in which the client feels comfortable making requests and offering constructive criticism. Too often, massage therapists cultivate their reputations as experts to such a degree that a client does not feel comfortable asking for what he or she wants. In order to effectively serve his or her clients, a therapist needs to be able to listen without judgment. Furthermore, the client's goals should always be the primary consideration when the therapist is making decisions.

Initial consultations

The initial consultation is perhaps the most important session in any therapeutic story because it establishes the relationship between the therapist and the client. In order to get the most out of this and any subsequent consultations, a therapist needs to be able to ask pertinent and effective questions. It is important for the therapist to establish an environment in which the client feels comfortable discussing his or her health. The therapist should remember that many clients will not have a vocabulary for what they are trying to express, and so the therapist should help draw their feelings out without dominating the conversation or distorting the client's point of view. A therapist should ask questions which give the client a chance to ruminate on his or her health history, and should seek to clarify any uncertain points by asking specific, objective questions.

Nonverbal communication

Because massage therapy is a profession concerned with touch, it is not surprising that some of the most important communication between massage therapists and clients is nonverbal. Nonverbal communication is not limited to touch, however. In order to establish a positive working relationship with a client, a massage therapist needs to communicate warmth and accessibility with his or her body language. A smile and a relaxed posture can be contagious and can help a client derive extra benefits from a massage session. Also, a therapist needs to consider the body language of a client and should tread lightly when a client seems peevish or defensive. Additionally, a client's body language will sometimes give the therapist information about his or her condition that the client cannot express through words.

Confidentiality

A massage therapist is required to respect the privacy of his or her clients by maintaining strict confidentiality standards. This means keeping client records in a secure location, and not sharing them with other practitioners without the permission of the client. In order to provide health information to another professional, even the client's doctor, you must receive permission from the client. Confidentiality can only be violated when it is obvious that there is an immediate danger to the client or some other person. In some rare cases, a client may not want to be recognized outside of the therapy environment. If you are in public and notice that a client seems to be avoiding you, do not make special efforts to attract the attention of the client.

History of Massage Practices

China

Ancient Chinese documents contain a wealth of information about massage, which apparently began to be practiced around 3000 B.C.E. The Chinese primarily used a system of touch called *anmo*, in which the flesh was manipulated with a combination of pressure and friction. Over time, Chinese massage therapists incorporated a practice known as *tui-na*, which literally means pushing and pulling. Tui-na was often combined with acupuncture, tai chi, and qigong. These massage techniques were part of a comprehensive health program, which also included exercise, nutrition, and medicinal herbs. The practice of acupuncture developed out of Chinese massage.

India, Japan, and Egypt

The ancient Indian text known as the *Ayur Veda* describes a system of hand rubbing and massage hygiene that was designed to improve circulation. Massage was incorporated into the system of stretches and exercises that evolved into yoga. This text was written between 1000 and 3000 B.C.E. In Japan, massage was not practiced until 600 A.D., at which time the technique of finger pressure known as *shiatsu* was developed. In Egypt, there are records of massage treatments dating back as far as 4000 B.C.E. Apparently, the members of the royal family received massage treatments to improve their health.

Ancient Greece

In ancient Greece, there was no mind/body duality; people assumed that, in order to have good mental health, it was necessary to be physically fit. The ancient Greeks revered massage therapy as an important part of health maintenance, along with exercise, nutrition, hygiene, and relaxation practices. The Greek baths offered full body massage treatment from trained masseuses. Athletes in particular were advised to partake in frequent massage to improve their performance on the field. The comprehensive program of health which incorporated exercise, hygienic practices, and massage was known as gymnastics. Both men and women partook in these activities.

Renaissance

After the fall of the Roman Empire, in which the ancient Greek customs of massage were practiced, the practice of massage therapy lay dormant for centuries. During the Renaissance (beginning roughly in 1450 A.D.), however, scholars began to promote the health benefits of regular massage therapy in their writings. The anatomical drawings completed by da Vinci and Vesalius gave massage therapists new insights into the musculature and physiology of the human body. Furthermore, doctors began to see the benefits of physically manipulating body tissue, which included stimulating circulation and improving vitality.

Per Henrik Ling

The Swedish physiologist Per Henrik Ling (1776-1839) is credited with ushering in the modern era of massage therapy. He developed the system of rhythmic symmetrical movements known as Swedish gymnastics, which incorporated muscular strength training, muscular endurance training, and flexibility exercises. Ling advocated repetitive movements incorporating both sides of the body, and gradually introduced a system of massage-like manipulations which came to be known as Swedish massage. Although these techniques bear little resemblance to the massage therapy practiced today, they are credited with reviving interest in massage therapy.

19th-century America

In the United States during the 19th century, a sudden increased interest in health led to a revival of massage techniques. American doctors and fitness instructors introduced the Swedish massage techniques, and added their own. The American physician John Harvey Kellogg (1842-1953) developed an extensive system of massage that paid attention to the various effects that massage had on the mechanics, reflexes, and metabolism of the body. His published work brought considerable attention to the health benefits of massage. Around the same time, the terminology of massage was being developed by a Dutch physician named Johann Mezger. Mezger is responsible for developing the important massage terms effleurage and pétrissage.

20th century

The 20th century has seen rapid developments in massage therapy, as well as a stunning growth in the number of distinct fields of practice. Many of the New Age movements of the 1960s endorsed massage as a means of unlocking human potential. More generally, though, doctors and exercise physiologists have continued to accumulate a body of research data describing the many positive effects of massage. Over the past 50 years, a number of professional organizations (including the American Massage Therapy Association) have been formed to advance the profession of massage therapy.

Swedish massage

Swedish massage is based on the physiological insights of Per Henrik Ling. Presently, it is the most common form of massage practiced in the United States. It involves the use of the hands, elbows, and lower arms. During a Swedish massage, the flesh of the client is kneaded and vigorously manipulated in order to increase circulation, promote relaxation, and diminish stress. Swedish massage includes several different kinds of strokes: effleurage (long, superficial strokes); pétrissage (kneading); tapotement (gentle beating); and rubbing. Research consistently shows that Swedish massage increases the flow of blood and lymphatic fluid throughout the body.

Practice Test

1. Which of the following accounts for approximately 16% of the human body?
   a.. Integumentary system.
   b. Skeletal system.
   c. Circulatory system.
   d. Respiratory system.

2. Which of the following systems is comprised of 206 individual organs?
   a. Integumentary system.
   b. Skeletal system.
   c. Circulatory system.
   d. Respiratory system.

3. Which of the following is comprised of smooth, voluntary, and cardiac tissues?
   a. Integumentary system.
   b. Skeletal system.
   c. Circulatory system.
   d. Muscular system.

4. What three main organs make up the nervous system?
   a. Brain, spinal cord, and ATP.
   b. Brain, skin, and nerves.
   c. Brain, spinal cord, and nerves.
   d. ATP, spinal cord, and nerves.

5. Which of the following systems acts like the nervous system, but with slower reaction time and longer-lasting effects?
   a. Integumentary system.
   b. Skeletal system.
   c. Cardiovascular system.
   d. Endocrine system.

6. Which of the following systems is a closed circuit whose main function is transportation through a network of vessels?
   a. Lymphatic system.
   b. Skeletal system.
   c. Cardiovascular system.
   d. Endocrine system.

7. Which of the following systems transports a whitish, watery fluid called lymph?
   a. Lymphatic system.
   b. Urinary system.
   c. Cardiovascular system.
   d. Endocrine system.

8. Which of the following systems produces waste in the kidney that moves to the ureters, and is stored in the urinary bladder?
   a. Lymphatic system.
   b. Urinary system.
   c. Respiratory system.
   d. Digestive system.

9. Which of the following systems functions as a means to rid the body of carbon dioxide?
    a. Lymphatic system.
    b. Urinary system.
    c. Respiratory system.
    d. Digestive system.

10. Which of the following systems include both the teeth and the pharynx?
    a. Lymphatic system.
    b. Urinary system.
    c. Respiratory system.
    d. Digestive system.

11. In the male reproductive system, what two organs make up the genitalia?
    a. The gonads and the penis.
    b. The penis and the scrotum.
    c. The prostate and the vas deferens.
    d. The scrotum and the gonads.

12. What organ is considered the female gonads?
    a. Ovaries
    b. Fallopian tube.
    c. Vagina
    d. Uterine.

13. Which of the following refer to the division of the cranial and sacral segments of the spinal cord?
    a. Craniosacral division.
    b. Sacralcranium division.
    c. Cranio and sacral aspects.
    d. Proprioception.

14. Which of the following types of membrane is found in closed cavities in the body?
    a. Cutaneous membranes.
    b. Serous membranes.
    c. Mucous membranes.
    d. Connective tissue membranes.

15. What information can the width of the epiphyseal plate tell a doctor?
    a. The strength of a bone.
    b. The estimated adult height of an individual.
    c. The probability of osteoporosis.
    d. The number of breaks a bone has had.

16. What is the purpose of the synergist in movement?
    a. Add support to the contracting prime mover.
    b. Counteract the prime mover.
    c. Relax as the antagonists contracts.
    d. Act as the main muscle in the movement.

17. Neurons are named for the direction they move. What are the three types neurons found in the body?
    a. Motor, Schwann, Interneurons.
    b. Sensory, Cranial, Interneurons.
    c. Sensory, Involuntary, Interneurons.
    d. Sensory, Motor, Interneurons.

18. What is the main mechanism behind the functioning of nonsteroid hormones?
    a. Negative feedback.
    b. Hypersecretion.
    c. Second messenger mechanism.
    d. Positive feedback.

19. What is the difference between the tunica externa in an artery compared to that in a vein?
    a. The tunica externa is thinner in arteries than in veins.
    b. The tunica externa is thicker in arteries than in veins.
    c. Arteries do not have a tunica externa.
    d. Veins do not have a tunica externa.

20. What percentage of the body moves lymph in to the thoracic duct?
    a. 100%.
    b. 75%.
    c. 50%.
    d. 25%.

21. What is the main function of the respiratory membrane?
    a. To line the respiratory tract with a layer of mucus.
    b. To act to separate air into the alveoli or the blood in the capillaries.
    c. To serve as a barrier to the outside air.
    d. To allow consistent oxygen flow into the blood stream.

22. Which of the following structures begins the process of digestion?
    a. Stomach.
    b. Small intestine.
    c. Teeth.
    d. Esophagus.

23. What is manipulated in the craniosacral system during a craniosacral therapeutic session?
    a. Dura mater.
    b. Interstitial fluid.
    c. Pia mater.
    d. Cerebrospinal fluid.

24. What occurs during the process of resorption?
    a. Fluid moves from the renal tubules into the blood stream.
    b. Fluid moves from the blood stream into the renal tubules.
    c. Fluid is filtered more than once.
    d. Elimination cannot occur and fluid is processed through the body again.

25. What is the term that refers to a body standing erect with hands at the sides and palms facing forward?
    a. Anatomical Position (western medicine).
    b. Anatomical Position (oriental medicine).
    c. Prone.
    d. Supine.

26. The plane that goes from top to bottom, which divides the body in left and right sides directly in the middle is referred to as which of the following?
    a. Sagittal.
    b. Frontal.
    c. Transverse.
    d. Midsagittal.

27. Which of the following are located in the dorsal cavity?
    a. The abdominopelvic cavity.
    b. The lungs.
    c. The thoracic cavity.
    d. None of the above.

28. Which of the following is not a major muscle of the head?
    a. Orbicularis oculi.
    b. Zygomaticus.
    c. Semimembranosus.
    d. Masseter.

29. Which muscle has an origin at the external occipital protuberance ligamentum nuchae and an insertion at the lateral third of clavicle acromion?
    a. Teres major.
    b. Latissimus dorsi.
    c. Trapezius.
    d. Teres minor.

30. Which of the following muscles has an action of medial rotation and adduction of the humerus?
    a. Teres major.
    b. Latissimus dorsi.
    c. Trapezius.
    d. Teres minor.

31. Which of the following is a depressor of the scapula?
    a. Upper trapezius.
    b. Upper pectoralis major.
    c. Lower trapezius.
    d. Serratus anterior.

32. What is occurring when a muscle contracts but no movement is produced?
    a. Twitch contraction.
    b. Tetanic contraction.
    c. Isotonic contraction.
    d. Isometric contraction.

33. What is occurring when a muscle experiences an involuntary quick movement?
    a. Twitch contraction.
    b. Tetanic contraction.
    c. Isotonic contraction.
    d. Isometric contraction.

34. What is the attachment which is on the more stationary bone?
    a. Tendon.
    b. Origin.
    c. Insertion.
    d. Bursae.

35. Which of the following connective tissues serve to anchor muscle to bone?
    a. Bursae.
    b. Tendon.
    c. Ligament.
    d. Sarcomere.

36. The iliopsoas and the adductor muscles work to move what part of the body?
    a. Head and neck.
    b. Arms.
    c. Thigh.
    d. Feet and ankles.

37. What function does the orbicularis oculi serve?
    a. Bring lips together.
    b. Elevates corners of lips.
    c. Close eyes.
    d. Opens eyes.

38. Which of the following joints are located in the skull?
    a. Synarthroses.
    b. Amphiarthroses.
    c. Diarthroses.
    d. There are no joints in the skull.

39. What is the most common type of join found in the human body?
    a. Synarthroses.
    b. Amphiarthroses.
    c. Diarthroses.
    d. Double joints.

40. A ball and socket joint can be found in what region of the body?
    a. Shoulder.
    b. Fingers.
    c. Spine.
    d. Knee.

41. Which of the following would a neurologist use to determine the specific point of damage on the spine?
    a. Spinal fracture test.
    b. Dermatomes.
    c. Motor reflex test.
    d. Meridians.

42. How many primary meridians make up the human body?
    a. 10
    b. 11.
    c. 12.
    d. 13.

43. Exposure to extreme heat, surgery, and illnesses are all examples of what on the body?
    a. Homeostasis.
    b. Disease.
    c. Stress.
    d. Heterostasis.

44. Which of the following typically results from a hypersecretion of glucocorticoids?
    a. Addison's disease.
    b. Cushing syndrome.
    c. Type I diabetes.
    d. Virilizing tumor.

45. Which of the following techniques would be used by an individual participating preparing to run in a marathon in 3 days?
    a. Carbohydrate loading.
    b. Protein loading.
    c. Glycogenesis.
    d. Antioxidant treatments.

46. What is required for muscles to contract?
    a. Myofilaments.
    b. Z-lines.
    c. ATP molecules.
    d. Actin.

47. What type of muscle contraction is occurring is a person is sitting up straight?
    a. Isotonic contraction.
    b. Tetanic contraction.
    c. Tonic contraction.
    d. Isometric contraction.

48. What type of movement is occurring in the angle between the forearm and humorous decreases?
    a. Flexion.
    b. Extension.
    c. Abduction.
    d. Adduction.

49. Moving your arms straight out to the sides requires what type of movement?
    a. Flexion.
    b. Extension.
    c. Abduction.
    d. Adduction

50. The downward motion of tapping your foot requires what type of movement?
    a. Rotation.
    b. Supination.
    c. Dorsiflexion.
    d. Plantar flexion.

51. Shaking your head "No" requires what type of movement?
    a. Rotation.
    b. Supination.
    c. Abduction.
    d. Adduction.

52. What must be stimulated in order to determine movement of the body?
    a. Muscles.
    b. Chakras.
    c. Proprioceptors.
    d. Bones.

53. Receptors that have some type of covering over their endings can be referred to as what?
    a. Closed-end receptors.
    b. Encapsulated.
    c. Unencapsulated.
    d. Sheathed bulb receptors.

54. In an individual with anorexia, what will the body rely on for energy once the fat stores are used up?
    a. Calcium.
    b. Carbohydrates.
    c. Proteins.
    d. Simple sugars.

55. What can occur from a deficiency of vitamin C?
    a. Scurvy.
    b. Night blindness.
    c. Nerve problems.
    d. Pernicious anemia.

56. Which of the following minerals, when deficient leads to fatigue and anemia?
    a. Calcium.
    b. Cobalt.
    c. Iodine.
    d. Copper.

57. If an individual has a deficiency in calories and protein, what disorder are they likely to have?
    a. Anorexia nervosa.
    b. Protein deficiency.
    c. Pro-caloric malnutrition.
    d. Protein-calorie malnutrition.

58. If a patient complains of pain in the left lumbar region, what organ is probably affected?
    a. Descending colon.
    b. Stomach.
    c. Liver.
    d. Kidneys.

59. Which function is responsible for maintaining equilibrium in the body?
    a. Homeostasis.
    b. Feedback loop.
    c. Biorhythm.
    d. Brain functions.

60. Which of the following has a phospholipid bilayer with proteins as its structure?
    a. Ribosomes.
    b. Mitochondria.
    c. Plasma membrane.
    d. Lysosomes.

61. If you get a paper cut on your finger, what type of tissue have you damaged?
    a. Epithelial tissue.
    b. Connective tissue.
    c. Muscle tissues.
    d. Nervous tissue.

62. Dr. Wright determined that 2-year-old Sammy will grow to be about 6-feet tall. What part of the bone did Dr. Wright look at to determine this number?
    a. Diaphysis.
    b. Articular cartilage.
    c. Epiphyseal plate.
    d. Endosteum.

63. When faced with a stressful situation, John's body began sweating. Why did this occur?
    a. Activation of the parasympathetic system. ↓
    b. Activation of the sympathetic system. ↑
    c. Activation of the endocrine system.
    d. Activation of the nervous system.

64. The ripple look of a toned stomach is the result of what type of muscle pattern?
    a. Multipennate.
    b. Fusiform.
    c. Strap.
    d. Tricipital.

Use the following to answer question 65:
    A new client comes in for a massage. She is a 35-year-old school teacher recommended by her doctor for massage. She is complaining about back and shoulder problems and states that she had shoulder surgery 8 months ago. As you read through the intake form, you also see that she is two months pregnant, has had massage in the past, and has migraine headaches. She also tells you that yesterday she fell while running and may have sprained her ankle but has not gone to the doctor.

65. Which of this client's medical situation is contraindicated for massage?
    a. Pregnancy.
    b. Shoulder surgery 8 months ago.
    c. Migraine headaches.
    d. Possible sprain.

66. If a massage therapist is calling a doctor to talk about a client with widespread pain, how would she describe this to the doctor?
    a. Pain all over.
    b. Fibromyalgia.
    c. Hypersensitivity.
    d. Hypo-muscle sensitivity.

67. Which of the following is probably not a part of the etiology of polycystic kidney disease?
    a. Cysts on the kidneys.
    b. Inherited.
    c. Mutation on PKD1 gene.
    d. 5% have end-stage renal disease.

Use the following to answer questions 68-69:
    A scientist studies the pattern of diseases and finds that a disease has spread from one country to the next on a large scale. Seeing that individuals with the disease experience chest pain, coughing blood, fever, chills, and weight loss, the scientist determines it is tuberculosis. Additionally, he notices that there are a large number of individuals who had silicosis prior to contracting tuberculosis. As the scientist discusses this situation with other doctors, they decide all healthcare workers must wear masks while near and treating these patients.

68. Why must healthcare workers wear masks when caring for these patients?
    a. It is an airborne illness.
    b. These patients emit a foul order.
    c. They are susceptible to other germs the healthcare workers may have.
    d. The air quality in the country may be very poor.

80

69. What would a healthcare worker refer to coughing blood, fever, chills, and weight loss as?
    a. Symptoms.
    b. Signs.
    c. Complaints.
    d. Idiopathic indications.

70. Which mood-altering chemicals are released during massage that could have a profound effect on an individual with depression?
    a. Serotonin.
    b. Estrogen.
    c. Adrenalin.
    d. Oxytocin.

71. Which of the following would be most appropriate for an individual with autism?
    a. No massage.
    b. Light, gentle strokes.
    c. Firm, purposeful touch.
    d. Hands and feet only.

72. How does a general relaxation massage benefit an individual with anxiety?
    a. Influences the automatic nervous system.
    b. Stimulates.
    c. Reduces hormones, causing anxiety.
    d. Anxiety is contraindicated.

73. What must a therapist be careful of in an individual with osteoporosis?
    a. Breaking a bone.
    b. Tearing a tendon.
    c. Causing emotional distress.
    d. Spreading the disease.

74. Which of the following refers to a signed document that gives the therapist permission to work on an individual?
    a. Right of refusal.
    b. Informed consent.
    c. Contract.
    d. Intake questionnaire.

Use the following to answer questions 75-78:
    You meet a new client and provide them with all the required paperwork, including an intake questionnaire and informed consent. After they have completed and signed the paper work, you review it and ask a few questions. You find out the individual has been under a lot of stress and emotional turmoil due to the recent loss of a spouse. They tell you a friend recommends massage as a way to relax. You can understand how they are feeling because you too recently lost a loved one. After the initial interview, you begin the massage. Your client asks for a gentle massage and lets you know they are not comfortable with massage on the face and gluts.

75. What would be occurring if your client began developing feelings for you beyond the client-therapist relationship and they state you are a lot like their deceased spouse?
    a. Violating legal boundaries.
    b. Violating personal boundaries.
    c. Transference.
    d. Countertransference.

76. What would be occurring if you developed feelings for your client beyond the client-therapist relationship?
  a. Violating legal boundaries.
  b. Violating personal boundaries.
  c. Transference.
  d. Countertransference.

77. How could you as a massage therapist cross your client's personal boundaries?
  a. Listen to your client throughout the massage.
  b. Massage their face.
  c. Listen and offer your assessment or opinion of their situation.
  d. Give them the name of a grief-counseling group.

78. How could you as a massage therapist cross legal or ethical boundaries?
  a. Listen to your client throughout the massage.
  b. Massage their face.
  c. Listen and offer your assessment or opinion of their situation.
  d. Give them the name of a grief-counseling group.

79. What is one way in which different types of healthcare workers, for example, a massage therapist and a physician, can communicate?
  a. Medical terminology.
  b. At conferences.
  c. Using notes to the client.
  d. Like normal people.

80. A massage therapist that rents a room from a spa would probably file their taxes under which category?
  a. Employee.
  b. Corporation.
  c. Independent contractor.
  d. Dependant.

81. How does a massage therapist maintain an individual's privacy throughout the massage?
  a. Keeping the door shut.
  b. Draping.
  c. Turning the lights on low.
  d. Massaging with your eyes closed.

82. Why would a therapist typically not massage the armpit?
  a. Endangerment site.
  b. The client is ticklish.
  c. The client does not shave.
  d. The client has body odor.

83. Suppose a client comes for a massage and states that his back pain began about 1 year ago, in terms of level of the condition, what would this back pain be considered?
  a. Acute.
  b. A sign.
  c. Chronic.
  d. A symptom.

84. What should you do if a client comes in for a massage and is ill?
   a. Send them home.
   b. Perform light massage.
   c. Refer them to a physician.
   d. Wear gloves.

85. A massage therapist talks about their client's illnesses and conditions, using names, at the dinner table each night. What has been violated?
   a. Confidentiality.
   b. Personal boundaries.
   c. Trust.
   d. Nothing.

86. Which of the following would help a therapist document their work on a client?
   a. HIPAA.
   b. S.O.A.P.
   c. ICD-9-CM.
   d. HPI.

87. Which of the following would contraindicate lymphatic massage?
   a. Congenital defect.
   b. Benign neoplasm.
   c. Malignant neoplasm.
   d. Chronic pain.

88. A sprain with 10% fiber tear would be classified as what type of sprain?
   a. Grade One.
   b. Grade Two.
   c. Grade Three.
   d. Grade Four.

89. A traumatic injury that results in 60% muscle fiber tear and swelling would be considered which of the following?
   a. First-degree strain.
   b. Second-degree strain.
   c. Third-degree strain.
   d. Fourth-degree strain.

90. Which type of bone fracture results in the bone being completely separated?
   a. Incomplete.
   b. Complete.
   c. Open.
   d. Fracture dislocation.

91. On which of the following types of headache would you consider performing trigger point therapy?
   a. Migraine.
   b. Cluster.
   c. Tension.
   d. Cervicogenic.

92. An individual would be experiencing which of the following if they were in shock due to loss of blood?
    a. Cardiogenic shock.
    b. Hypovolemic shock.
    c. Neurogenic shock.
    d. Anaphylactic shock.

93. Which of the following is not considered an upper respiratory infection?
    a. Rhinitis.
    b. Pharyngitis.
    c. Laryngitis.
    d. Bronchitis.

94. If an individual states that they have hypernatremia, what is happening in their body?
    a. Potassium imbalance.
    b. Sodium imbalance.
    c. Calcium imbalance.
    d. Dehydration.

95. Which of the following is not a purpose of massage?
    a. To increase cell metabolism.
    b. To heal illness.
    c. To increase ROM.
    d. To relieve pain.

96. Breaking up adhesions using petrissage would be considered what type of effect on the body?
    a. Mechanical.
    b. Physiological.
    c. Psychological.
    d. Pain-relieving.

97. On what does lymph rely to be moved through the body?
    a. Blood flow.
    b. Voluntary muscles.
    c. Involuntary muscles.
    d. Massage.

98. What is one result of over stimulation of the nervous system to muscles?
    a. Relaxation.
    b. Pain.
    c. Spasm.
    d. Injury.

99. Which of the following is typically the first stroke to begin a massage?
    a. Petrissage.
    b. Friction.
    c. Effleurage.
    d. Tapotement.

100. Which of the following strokes can enhance fluid movement of deeper tissue?
    a. Petrissage.
    b. Friction.
    c. Effleurage.
    d. Tapotement.

101. Which of the following best describes abnormal restrictions to joint movements?
    a. Reduced range of motion.
    b. Reduced joint movement.
    c. Passive joint movement.
    d. Active joint movement.

102. Which of the following is indicated for massage?
    a. Asthma.
    b. Abdominal aneurysm.
    c. Bursitis.
    d. Edema.

103. Which of the following best describes an effect of hydrotherapy that affects the entire body?
    a. Local effect.
    b. Systemic effect.
    c. Reflex effect.
    d. Thermal effect.

104. Which of the following refer to the study of movement?
    a. Biomechanics.
    b. Synergists.
    c. Kinesiology.
    d. Massage therapy.

105. In Kinesiology, which of the following aspects of an assessment would include passive ROM?
    a. History.
    b. Observation.
    c. Palpation.
    d. Specialized testing.

106. Which of the following organelles are found only in the small intestine?
    a. Cilia.
    b. Flagella.
    c. Microvilli.
    d. Centrioles.

107. In terms of an active transport system, which of the following move molecules against the concentration gradient?
    a. Phagocytosis.
    b. Pinocytosis.
    c. Permease System.
    d. Filtration.

Use the following vignette to answer questions 108-111:
    Newly licensed massage therapist Amy immediately opens an office. She figures she will figure out the business aspect of owning a business as so goes. She has named her massage business "The Healing Touch" and has created signs, advertising materials, and business cards with a logo. She is on time for all massage appointments, keeps the waiting room neat and stocked with information about massage, and has her license displayed on the wall. The only records Amy keeps are the client records and she notes the date and amount paid for all massages from that client. Amy has purchased insurance including Property Damage, Bodily Injury Liability, and Malpractice insurance. Her insurance agent also suggests that she purchase Business and Personal Property Loss and Disability insurance, but Amy declines.

108. If Amy's office undergoes a flood, leading to $1,000 in damage, why will she have to pay out-of-pocket expenses?
    a. She did not purchase enough Property Damage insurance.
    b. She did not purchase Business & Personal Property Loss insurance.
    c. Floods are not covered under any insurance.
    d. The damage did not meet her deductible.

109. A client fell in the waiting room of Amy's office, why does Amy feel secure that she is covered in this incident?
    a. She has Malpractice insurance.
    b. She has Property Damage and Bodily Injury Liability insurance.
    c. She rents the office, so the landlord is responsible.
    d. The injury did not occur during the massage, so it is the client's responsibility.

110. In the above vignette, what, concerning the business aspect, does Amy neglect to do?
    a. Create a professional image.
    b. Purchase Disability insurance.
    c. Develop a business plan.
    d. Advertise in the newspaper.

111. What has Amy created by developing a logo and marketing materials?
    a. A business plan.
    b. Professional image.
    c. Additional bills.
    d. A sound marketing plan.

112. A client comes in for a massage and complains that due to a back injury, they currently rely on their family members to take care of their home. To whom might you refer this client in order to increase their quality of life and independence?
    a. Chiropractor.
    b. Acupuncturist.
    c. Occupational Therapist.
    d. Physical Therapist.

113. What are the three steps to take for a primary survey when faced with an individual who may not be breathing?
    a. Airway, breathing, circulation.
    b. Clear the area, check breathing, check for neck injury.
    c. Airway, clear the area, circulation.
    d. Call 911, clear the area, check Breathing.

114. Which of the following is the most efficient standing position for a massage therapist?
    a. Symmetric standing.
    b. Asymmetric standing.
    c. Knees slightly bent.
    d. Knees locked.

115. Which of the following refers to a passive joint movement?
    a. Osteokinematic movement.
    b. Arthrokinematic movement.
    c. Hinge movement.
    d. Joint movement.

116. What is the point at which injury would occur to a joint?
    a. Physiologic barrier.
    b. Pathologic barrier.
    c. Anatomic barrier.
    d. Range of motion.

117. For which massage therapy setting would it be most beneficial for a therapist to know and understand various dysfunctions of the body?
    a. Private practice.
    b. Medical office.
    c. Spa.
    d. Chiropractor's office.

118. On what bodily system does hydrotherapy focus?
    a. Integumentary.
    b. Muscle.
    c. Autonomic nervous.
    d. Respiratory.

119. Which of the following massage techniques could leave the client feeling fatigued and listless for up to 48 hours after the massage?
    a. Hydrotherapy.
    b. Swedish massage.
    c. Lymphatic drainage.
    d. Reflexology.

120. Which of the following is contraindicated for lymphatic drainage?
    a. Simple edema.
    b. Low blood pressure.
    c. High blood pressure.
    d. Traveler's edema.

Answers and Explanations

1. A: The Integumentary system, also known as the skin, accounts for approximately 16% of the human body. In the average adult, the skin alone weighs approximately 20 pounds. While this system is also referred to as the skin, it is important to note that the hair, nails, and sweat and oil glands are also included in this system. Within this system, particularly in the skin, lie sense organs that allow a person to feel temperature, pain, and pressure. This main function of the Integumentary system is to provide protection to the other organs and tissues in the body, as well as to serve as temperature regulator and a means to synthesize various chemicals.

2. B: The Skeletal system is composed of 206 bones that provide the structure and support for the human body. In addition to the bones, within this system are tissue, cartilage, and ligaments that provide the connections and support for the bones themselves. Within the skeletal system, there are two main parts, which include the axial skeleton and the appendicular skeleton. The Axial skeleton includes the bones of the skull, the ribs, and the neck and spine. The appendicular skeleton includes the bones in the shoulder, arm and hands, pelvis, legs, and feet. These two divisions of the skeletal system are attached at the pectoral girdle, the group including the scapula and the clavicle.

3. D: The Muscular system is made up of three different muscle types including the smooth muscles, cardiac muscles, and voluntary muscles. The smooth muscles also referred to as involuntary muscles can be found in the colon, stomach, and eyes. These muscles work constantly and do not require conscious thought to perform. Voluntary muscles also referred to as skeletal muscles, take conscious effort in order to be put into action. These muscles are found on the skeleton and assist in movement. Cardiac muscles are found in the heart and are involuntary.

4. C: The nervous system includes the brain, spinal cord, and the nerves. This system serves a number of functions including communication from the brain to the body, control, and integration. All processes completed by the nervous system are completed through nerve impulses that move quickly through the body to the brain, relaying various messages. These messages will depend on which stimuli are present. For example, if you touch something hot, the nerves in your hand will relay a message to the brain based on the stimuli, the brain will process and response by sending nerve impulses back to the hand, telling the hand that it is hot.

5. D: The Endocrine system functions much like the nervous system in that it communicates, integrates, and controls. The way this system accomplishes these functions is by secreting hormones throughout the body through a series of ducts and glands. Some of the main activities the endocrine system controls and regulates include growth, metabolism, reproduction, etc. Glands within this system are ductless and are located throughout the body. For examples, in the brain are the pituitary gland and the hypothalamus, in the neck are the thyroid and the parathyroid glands, the thymus gland in the thoracic cavity, and just below in the abdominal cavity are the adrenal glands and the pancreas.

6. C: The Cardiovascular system is made up of the heart, arteries, veins, and capillaries that transport nutrients, oxygen, carbon dioxide, and waste through the blood to all sections of the body. This closed-circuit system also serves to regulate body temperature and some specialized cells of the cardiovascular system assist with the immune system. Also called the circulatory system, blood travels through the heart, leaving it by way of arteries and continues through the arterioles, capillaries, venules, and veins. The blood then returns to the heart through veins. In addition to this systemic circulation, pulmonary circulation is the process for transporting blood to the lungs; hepatic portal circulation transports blood through the liver, and fetal circulation transports blood to and from a fetus.

7. A: The Lymphatic system transports lymph and is composed of the lymph nodes, lymphatic vessels, and other lymphatic organs such as the tonsils, spleen, and the thymus gland. Lymph contains various fatty molecules, proteins, and lymphocytes. It must be noted that there are no red blood cells within the Lymphatic system. While the lymph is transported through its own lymphatic vessels, this material will eventually travel through ducts in to the main blood stream. Two common areas in the body where lymph can be found include the armpit and the groin, were there are large collections of lymph nodes.

8. B: The Urinary system is composed of the kidneys, ureters, the bladder, and the urethra. Within this system, it is the kidney's role to clear the blood that is transported into this organ. This blood, before it is cleaned, contains waste from metabolized food. Once waste, or urine, is produced in the kidneys, it travels out of this organ in to the ureters and is stored in the bladder. As the urine leaves the body it will flow from the bladder through the urethra. Other organs that serve to rid the body of waste include the intestines, skin, and lungs.

9. C: The Respiratory system rids the body of carbon dioxide. Within the system are the nose, pharynx, larynx, trachea, bronchi, and the lungs. This system can be further broken down in to the upper respiratory system (nose, pharynx, and larynx) and the lower respiratory system (trachea, bronchi, and the lungs). Air enters the respiratory system through the nose travels through the pharynx in to the larynx to the trachea and the bronchi into the lungs, into alveoli. Alveoli are small, thin sacs where oxygen is exchanged for carbon dioxide and the carbon dioxide leaves the body. In cold climates, the air is warmed in the upper respiratory system.

10. D: The Digestive or gastrointestinal system included the teeth and the pharynx. Additionally, this system includes the mouth, esophagus, stomach, small intestine, large intestine, rectum, anal canal, salivary glands, tongue, live, gallbladder, pancreas and the appendix. This system is divided in to two groups, which include primary organs (mouth, esophagus, pharynx, stomach, small intestine, large intestine, rectum, anal canal) and accessory organs (teeth, salivary glands, tongue, liver, gallbladder, pancreas, and the appendix). As food passes through the digestive tract, important nutrients will be absorbed by the body and the remaining will exit the body as waste product.

11. B: The penis and the scrotum make up the male genitalia in the male reproductive system. Within this system, the genitalia are considered supporting organs. Additionally, in the male reproductive system the gonads, or testes, are responsible for sperm production. The vas deferens and the prostate also act as accessory organs in the process of reproduction. During reproduction, the sperm travels from the testes through the vas deferens and other genital ducts through the urethra and out of the body. In this process, the prostate is responsible for producing nutrient-filled fluid that assists in reproduction.

12. A: Within the female reproductive system, the ovaries are the female gonads. Eggs are produced in the ovaries and travel through the fallopian tubes and will attach to the wall of the uterus if fertilized. Other organs in the female reproductive system include the vagina, vulva, and the mammary glands. The vagina is a tube approximately 10-cm long and is composed of involuntary muscle. It is located in between the balder and the rectum in the pelvic cavity. The vagina is also referred to as the birth canal. The vulva is the external female genitalia. Finally the mammary glands, located in the breast, are also considered external sex organs.

13. A: The Craniosacral division is the nerves of the parasympathetic division that lead off from the cranial and the sacral segments of the spinal cord. This system results in an opposite response to the sympathetic systems, and includes the contraction of the pupils and the return to a normal heart rate. In addition to these effects, the craniosacral system as a whole has an impulse called the craniosacral impulse. This impulse can be palpated through slow and steady body work. The impulse is the rhythm of the individual's body and will vary from person to person.

14. B: Serous membranes are found in the closed cavities of the body. This type of membrane is classified as an epithelial membrane and is made up of two layers. This top layer is the squamous epithelium and the bottom layer is connective tissues called the basement membrane. Additionally, these membranes are named according to where in the body they are located and what they cover, and more specifically, when covering the wall of a cavity it is termed a parietal portion and when covering an organ this membrane is termed the visceral portion. Serous membranes within the thoracic cavity are referred to as pleura, and those within the abdominal cavity are referred to at peritoneum. Therefore, the serous membrane that covers the wall of the abdominal cavity is called the parietal peritoneum, covering the organs within the abdominal cavity referred to as the visceral peritoneum. Those covering the lining of the thoracic cavity are referred to as the parietal pleura, whereas those covering the organs within the thoracic cavity are called visceral pleura.

15. B: The width of the epiphyseal plate can provide information for an estimate of the adult height of an individual. The epiphyseal plate is located between the epiphyses and the diaphysis within bone and as children, this is a cartilage substance. This estimate may be made when the individual is a child, prior to ossification. A common technique for this estimation is obtaining an x-ray of a child's bones, often the wrist, and determining if and how much of the epiphyseal plate is cartilage. As the child grows, this plate will completely transform into bone, at which point the individual will stop growing.

16. A: As a muscle moves, the synergist provides support to the prime mover. Both the synergist and the prime mover muscles contract while the antagonist muscles relax. Therefore, the movement of pulling your forearm up requires your biceps brachii to be the prime movers and the bicep brachialis serve as the synergists. The triceps are the antagonist of the movement because they are required to relax in order to stretch out. As the forearm is moved back down in a straight position, the role of these muscles is reversed and the triceps becomes the prime mover and the biceps brachii the antagonist.

17. D: Sensory neurons provide information to the brain from various parts of the body. This type of neuron is also referred to as afferent neurons. Motor neurons, also referred to as efferent neurons, send signals and information from the brain to either muscle or glandular epithelial tissue. These neurons send signals that tell the various parts of the body what to do. Interneurons act as connecting neurons as they send information from the motor neurons to the sensory neurons. Together, these three types of neurons create a loop-type system of information transfer. As an example of this process, if an individual touches something hot, that information will be sent up to the brain through the sensory neurons; once the brain processes the information, it is sent back through motor neurons. The interneurons come into play when information must be passed from the sensory to the motor neurons and vice versa.

18. C: The second messenger mechanism is the main mechanism of functioning for nonsteroid hormones. For this process, a first messenger is required; commonly a protein hormone which will attach to a specific receptor site on the cell membrane. Once the connection between the protein hormone and the cell receptor site has been accomplished, chemical reaction occurs and activates the second messengers, which are in the cell. Once the second messengers are activated, then the hormone can carry out its specific function. This process is a form of communication between the hormones and the cells. A common example of this process can be demonstrated by the hormone adenosine monophosphate, which is a second messenger that provides the cell with necessary information for activity.

19. A: The tunica externa is the outermost layer of both an artery and a vein, and is thinner in arteries. This layer is composted of connective tissue, and its primary function is that of support and reinforcement of the artery or vein to prevent bursting under the pressure of blood flow. In addition to this layer, arteries and veins also have a tunica media, responsible for the regulation of blood pressure, and tunica intima, a smooth film lining arteries and veins that prevents unintentional blood clotting. Unique to veins are the semilunar valves located within the tunica intima. These valves prevent backflow of blood as it travels back to the heart.

20. B: Approximately 75% of the body dumps its lymph into the thoracic duct. The thoracic duct is located on the left subclavian vein and is the largest lymphatic vessel in the body. Lymph for all parts of the body except the upper right extremity flows through the thoracic duct. In addition to the thoracic duct, the right lymphatic duct is located on the right subclavian vein. Lymph from the right sides of the head, neck, chest, and right arm enter into the right lymphatic duct. All lymph flows in one direction and eventually enters back into the blood stream to be discarded as waste. Additionally, a structure in the abdomen, called the cistern chili, acts as a storage area for lymph traveling toward the thoracic duct.

21. B: The respiratory membrane acts to separate air into the alveoli, or the blood in the capillaries. This membrane can be found lining the wall of the alveoli, which are small sacs that fill with air located at the end of the bronchioles. The respiratory membrane consists of various layers including the alveolar wall, interstitial fluid, and the pulmonary capillary wall. The alveolar wall is comprised of epithelial cells, while the pulmonary capillary wall is made up of endothelial cells. The process of oxygen and carbon dioxide travelling across the respiratory membrane is diffusion.

22. C: Digestion begins in the mouth with the teeth. The teeth serve digestion by breaking food down for further processing. While the mouth is considered a main organ within the digestive system, the teeth are accessory organs. The tongue, also an accessory organ, assists the teeth in this initial breakdown of food. From the mouth, food will travel down the pharynx to the esophagus, then to the stomach, the small intestine, the large intestine, the rectum, and finally the anal canal. As the food moves through this system, various chemical reactions occur and food is metabolized as essential nutrients are removed and distributed or stored in the body as needed.

23. D: Cerebrospinal fluid is manipulated during a craniosacral therapeutic session. This fluid can be found between the dura mater, the arachnoid membrane, and the pia mater. These three layers of membrane make up the meningeal system. More specifically, the dura mater is the outermost membrane and functions as waterproof protection. The arachnoid membrane is the middle layer, and provides the necessary lubrication for the outer- and innermost membranes of this system to easily glide. Finally, the pia mater is the innermost membrane that lines the brain and spinal cord. Because the cerebrospinal fluid serves as lubrication between these membrane layers, if this fluid is not flowing freely through the craniosacral system, then pain may result.

24. A: With the process of resorption, fluid moves from the renal tubules into the blood stream. Common substances that undergo the process of resorption include water, proteins, sodium, and other essential nutrients. Resorption begins at the proximal convoluted tubules through the loop of Henle, through the distal convoluted tubules and into the collecting tubules. Resorption occurs through osmosis, and nearly 99% of water is resorbed on a daily basis. Additionally, one nutrient, glucose, is also resorbed. The body's inability to resorb glucose results in a condition referred to as glycosuria, or glucose in the urine, which is a sign of diabetes mellitus.

25. A: The Anatomical Position, according to western medicine, is achieved when the body standing erect with hands at the sides and palms facing forward. In addition, the head and feet also face forward. This universal position allows communication between professionals in the healthcare industry. Using the anatomical position as a reference point, we are able to discuss and locate various parts of the body. In terms of referencing the body using this position, anatomical directions include superior (toward the head) and inferior (away from the head); anterior (front) and posterior (back); medial (toward the midline) and lateral (toward the side); proximal (toward the trunk) and distal (away from the trunk); and superficial (near the surface) and deep (away from the surface).

26. D: The midsagittal is the plane that goes from top to bottom, which divides the body in left and right sides directly in the middle. This should not be confused with the sagittal plane, which divides the body in left and right sides but does not do so directly down the middle of the body or organ. Other planes that are used to determine and discuss a specific location of the body include frontal, running side to side and dividing the body into front and back, and transverse, running horizontally, dividing the body into top and bottom.

27. D: None of the above. The abdominopelvic cavity and the thoracic cavity are divisions of the ventral cavity. The lungs are contained within the thoracic cavity. The dorsal cavity consists of the cranial cavity and spinal canal.

28. C: The semimembranosus is not a major muscle of the head, but is in fact a muscle of the hamstring group, with an insertion at the tibia and origin at the ischium and functions to flex the knee. The Orbicularis oculi is located above the eye, with an insertion and origin at the maxilla and functions to closes the eye. The Zygomaticus is located at the cheek with an insertion at the angle of the mouth and upper lip and an origin at the Zygomatic arch and functions to elevate the corners of the mouth. Finally, the Masseter is located at the jaw with an insertion at the mandible and an origin at the Zygomatic arch and functions to close the mouth.

29. C: The trapezius has an origin at the external occipital protuberance ligamentum nuchae and an insertion at the lateral third of clavicle acromion. The trapezius also has an origin at the C7-T12 spinous process and two additional insertions at the spine of the scapula and the root of the spine of the scapula. The trapezius is a triangular shaped muscle and is the most superficial muscle in the back. The action of the trapezius is elevation and upward rotation of the scapula, and retraction of the scapula. This muscle lies superior to the latissimus dorsi, and the teres major and minor.

30. B: The latissimus dorsi has an action of medial rotation and adduction of the humerus. This muscle also has an origin at the thoracolumbar aponeurosis, the lower six thoracic spinous processes, the iliac crest and the sacrum, the lower 4 ribs, and the inferior angle of the scapula. The insertion of the latissimus dorsi is at the bicipital groove of the humerus. This muscle is the widest muscle in the back and is very useful for activities that require a lot of power such as swimming. In addition to the action of rotation, the latissimus dorsi is responsible for extension.

31. C: The lower trapezius is a depressor of the scapula.

32. D: An isometric contraction occurs when a muscle contracts but no movement is produced. Isometric is a Greek word meaning "equal measure." As it pertains to muscle movement and contraction, if a muscle shortens, then it will move. However, in this type of muscle contraction the length in the relaxed state is the same, or equal to the length of the muscle in the contracted state. What is occurring within the muscle during an isometric contraction is that the muscle tension increases. This type of contraction can be accomplished by pushing or pulling on a stationary object.

33. A: A twitch contraction is an involuntary, quick movement. This type of muscle contraction typically occurs in response to a stimulus; for example, a fly landing on your arm or touching something too hot or too cold. Research on muscle contractions such as twitches has been able to isolate individual muscles and cause these individual muscle fibers to twitch. However, in real-life movements, a twitch will not occur on an isolated muscle fiber due to the all-or-none response. This muscle response is one in which either all the fibers of a muscle move, or none of them move.

34. B: The origin is the muscle attachment on the more stationary bone. Every muscle will have an origin and there are a number of muscles that have more than one origin. The tendons, on the other hand, are tissue that connects the muscle to the bone. Tendons will be found at both the insertion and the origin of the muscle. The insertion is the part of the muscle that is attached on the more movable part. Finally the bursae are sacs filled with fluid located between the tendon and the bone. These fluid-filled sacs help with movement by providing a lubricant called the synovial fluid.

35. B: Tendons anchor the muscle to the bone. Tendons are made up of dense connective tissue so that the muscle firmly attaches to bone. Tendons are further protected by tendon sheaths. These tendon sheaths are lined with a synovial membrane that provides lubrication to the tendon in order to allow for easy movement. The bursae can be found between some tendons and the bone and serve to provide lubrication to decrease friction between the tendon and bone. Without the tendon sheaths and the bursae, movement would be painful and very difficult, because the tendons would not be able to easily move, and the friction between the bone and the tendon would result in tearing.

36. C: The iliopsoas and the adductor muscles serve to move the lower extremities. Specifically, the iliopsoas has an origin at the ilium and vertebrae and an insertion at the femur. This muscle flexes the thigh and the trunk of the body. Other muscles that move the thigh or the trunk of the body include the sartorius (flexes thigh and rotates legs) and the gluteus maximus (extends thigh). The adductor muscles are a group that includes the adductor longus, gracilis, and the pectineus, all of which adduct the thigh. All three adductor muscles have an origin at the pubis, while the adductor longus and pectineus have an insertion at the femur and the gracilis has an insertion at the tibia.

37. C: The orbicularis oculi closes the eyes. This muscle has an origin and insertion at the maxilla and the frontal bone, and therefore circles the eye. Another muscle that moves the eyes is the frontal muscle with an origin at the occipital bone and insertion at the eyebrow, this muscle raises the eyebrows. The muscles that move the eyes are important for facial expressions. While these muscles move the eye brows and eye lids, there are a number of muscles in the skull that move the eyeball itself. These include the medial, lateral, superior, and inferior rectus muscles, and the superior and inferior oblique muscles.

38. A: The skull contains synarthroses joints, also referred to as suture because of the suture-like appearance. In newborns these joints are not fully formed, resulting in the soft spot on the top of the head which is fibrous tissue. As the child grows, the bones close. These joints are immobile because connective tissue has grown between the bones. While synarthroses joints are often discussed in terms of having mo movement, those in the skull do have slight movement caused by the ebb and flow of spinocranial fluid. In craniosacral therapy, the bones in the skull are palpated and the therapist can feel the movement of these bones.

39. C: Diorthoses joints are the most common type of joint in the human body. These joints move freely. All diorthoses joints have three common structures, which include the joint capsule, joint cavity, and cartilage covering the ends of the two adjoining bones. These structures are made up of connective tissues and synovial membranes that allow the joint to move in one or more directions. The type of movement a diorthoses joint has will depend on its location within the body and the specific joint type. Joint types include ball and socket, hinge, pivot, saddle, gliding, and condyloid.

40. A: The joint in the shoulder is a ball and socket joint. This type of joint allows full movement of the shoulder which includes side to side, up and down, and in a circular motion. With ball and socket joints, the end of one bone is shaped like a ball and the end of the other bones is a concave, cup-like shape. These two bones fit snuggly together with a synovial membrane separating them to reduce friction and allow easy movement. When a joint is "popped out of socket" this is referring to this ball and socket joint, when the ball end comes out of the socket end.

41. B: Neurologists use dermatomes to determine the exact location of a spinal injury. Dermatomes refer to specific locations on the skin surface that are connected to only one nerve. Looking at a dermatome map of the body, one can see that the skin surface is divided into 5 segments, or dermatomes; cervical, thoracic, lumbar, sacral, and coccygeal. Within each of these segments are further divisions or layers that connect to a specific nerve. More specifically, there are 8 cervical, 12 thoracic, 5 lumbar, 5 sacral, and one coccygeal nerve; therefore each segment has the corresponding subdivisions.

42. C: There are 12 primary meridians in the human body including the lung, colon, stomach, spleen, heart, intestine, triple warmer, pericardium, urinary bladder, kidney, gallbladder, and liver meridians. Each point of these meridians corresponds to a location, function, and time in the body, and all primary meridians correspond to an internal organ. In oriental medicine, meridians carry the flow of Qi to all parts of the body. The flow of Qi is as follows: note the time in parentheses refers to the time of activity for that organ: lungs (3:00 AM-5:00 AM), large intestine (5:00 AM-7:00 AM), stomach (7:00 AM-9:00 AM), spleen (9:00 AM-11:00 AM), heart (11:00 AM-1:00 PM), small intestine (1:00 PM-3:00 PM), urinary bladder (3:00 PM-5:00 PM), kidney (5:00 PM-7:00 PM), pericardium (7:00 PM-9:00 PM), triple warmer (9:00 PM-11:00 PM), gallbladder (11:00 PM-1:00 AM), and liver (1:00 AM-3:00 AM).

43. C: Stress is the condition in which the body is not in balance. Stressors on the body can range and include physical or mental stimuli. During stress glucocorticoid production and release is increased by the adrenal cortex. This process is the first step in the stress response. Once glucocorticoid concentrations are elevated in the body, there is an increase in the amount of fats and proteins that are metabolized atrophy in the thymus, and the inflammatory response becomes inhibited. From here other stress responses are put into action until the body once again reaches homeostasis, or balance.

44. B: Cushing syndrome typically results from a hypersecretion of glucocorticoids. This syndrome is characterized by physical abnormalities such as moon-face and buffalo hump. These abnormalities are cause because of an abnormal redistribution of fat causing the face or upper back, respectively to be larger and more rounded than normal. Another common symptom of this syndrome is an increased production of testosterone leading to the appearance of male secondary sexual characteristics. This syndrome is more common in women and individuals with Cushing have higher than normal blood sugar levels and frequent infections. The physical abnormalities of this syndrome can be corrected with surgery.

45. A: Carbohydrate loading would be the most beneficial nutritional practice or technique for an individual preparing for a marathon. Carbohydrate loading is the intake of a large amount of carbohydrates for storage in the body, specifically, in skeletal muscle fibers. When athletes consume a high carbohydrate diet, they are able to store up to two times as many carbohydrates as normal. This additional energy will allow them to sustain physical activity for a longer period. As energy is needed, the body takes the stored carbohydrates and processes them through glucose catabolism, which has three stages: (1) glycolysis; (2) citric acid cycle; and (3) electron transfer system.

46. C: Muscle contraction requires energy or ATP molecules. With a muscle contraction, all parts of the muscle are involved, otherwise known as an all-or-nothing response. Specifically, the muscle is composed of fibers with thick and thin myofilaments that produce proteins, myosin and actin, respectively, upon contraction. The action of a contracting muscle can be observed by looking at the sarcomeres. As the muscle contrasts, the distance between the z-lines of the sarcomeres shortens, whereas when the muscle relaxes, the distance increases. Thick and thin myofilaments slide toward each other, overlapping during muscle contraction. This is also referred to as the sliding filament model.

47. C: In a tonic contraction, there is no muscle movement. However, the muscles do serve to support the body. A tonic contraction will occur anytime an individual is in an upright position. Another way to describe this type of contraction is posture. Individuals with good posture have strong muscles that are also properly aligned with other parts of the body; the opposite is true for individuals with poor posture. The muscles specifically involved in maintaining posture are back and neck muscles, because gravity tends to pull the head and trunk of the body down.

48. A: Flexion occurs when there is a decrease in the angle between two bones. In addition to the decrease in the angle, during flexion, there is a decrease in the length of the prime mover and an increase in the length of the antagonist associated with the bones. In this example, when the angle between the forearm and the humorous decreases, the length of the bicep decreases while the triceps increase in length. Similar to flexing the arm, one can also flex the leg in which one would bend the leg back at the knee, shortening the hamstring muscle group and lengthening the quadriceps.

49. C: Abduction is a movement away from the midline. By moving your arms straight out to the sides and away from the midline, you are abducting your arms. Muscles involved in this type of movement include the deltoid as the prime mover and rotator cuff muscles as the synergists. In order for abduction to occur, the deltoid must contract. Additionally, the glenohumeral joint is also involved. The opposite movement to abduction is adduction. Adduction is the movement toward the midline. When you bring your arms back down to your body, adduction occurs.

50. D: Plantar flexion results in the toes pointing downward. Plantar flexion is also required to move into a position where you are standing on your toes. This movement will increase the degree of the angle between the top of the foot and the ankle. The primary muscles involved in plantar flexion include the gastrocnemius, soleus, plantaris, flexor hallucis longus, flexor digitorum longus, and the tibialis posterior. The lateral muscles involved in this movement include the peroneus longus and peroneus brevis. The opposite movement is dorsiflexion, which results in the toes pointing upward and decreased the degree of the angle between the top of the foot and the ankle.

51. A: Rotation is the movement that occurs when shaking your head "no." This movement occurs around a longitudinal axis. The main joint type in the neck that allows this movement is a condyloid joint. Other types of rotation include internal rotation, also referred to as media rotation. Internal rotation is a rotation toward the midline. For example, you can rotate your shoulder or hip toward your midline. External rotation, or lateral rotation, is the movement of rotation away from the midline. Rotating your hip out so your toes point away from the midline is an example of external rotation.

52. C: Proprioceptors are receptors found between tendons and muscles as well as deep within the skeleton that provide the brain with information about body position or movement. These receptors are enclosed. When there is trauma to a proprioceptor, it could result in permanent damage, leading to the loss of feeling of the muscles. Two important proprioceptors include the Golgi tendons and muscle spindles. Golgi tendons are located at the junction of tendons and muscles and detect tension the muscle. Muscle spindles located in all skeletal muscles detect the length of a muscle.

53. B: Receptors are often distinguished by whether or not they are encapsulated (covered) or unencapsulated (free or naked). There are six main encapsulated receptors. Meissner's corpuscles located on the skin, fingertips, and lips and detect very fine touches and low frequency vibrations. Ruffini's corpuscles are also located at the dermal layer of the skin and the subcutaneous tissues of the fingers and detect both touch and pressure. The Pacinian corpuscles are located at various levels of tissues at joints, the mammary glands, and external genitalia and detect pressure and high frequency vibrations. Krause's end-bulbs are located in the skin, lips, eyelids, and external genitalia and detect touch and cold. Golgi tendons and muscle spindles, located in skeletal muscles detect muscle tension and length.

54. C: Anorexia is an illness in which the individual starves themselves. In these cases the body will compensate for the lack of nutrients and use up all available resources. This begins with the use of all stored fat throughout the body. Following this, the body will begin to use up its protein stores in order to provide itself with energy. During this process, the protein molecules will go through catabolism and the amino acids making up these proteins will be broken down and converted into glucose which then begins the citric acid cycle. Because the body needs proteins for survival, when the body uses these proteins solely for energy, death may occur.

55. A: An individual with a vitamin C deficiency may develop scurvy. Scurvy is characterized by the inability to make and maintain collagen fibers which is necessary for connective tissues. Common physical symptoms of scurvy include skin spots, spongy gums, and bleeding. Prior to modern day technologies and knowledge about the importance of vitamins, this disease was very common among sailors who may not have had efficient access to the fruits and vegetables that provide vitamin C. While if untreated, scurvy can be fatal, individuals with this disease can make full recoveries with the intake of vitamin C.

56. D: Copper is an essential mineral. Individuals deficient in copper may experience fatigue and anemia. Adequate amounts of copper can be found in seafood, organ meats, and legumes. Copper's primary function in the body with regard to metabolism is to extract energy from the citric acid cycle of catabolism as well as during the production of blood. In addition to these functions, copper also serves to provide the blood with oxygen and maintain healthy hair color. While copper can be obtained from various foods, the body is also able to absorb copper through the skin and many individuals have found wearing copper jewelry, particularly bracelets, beneficial for ailments such as arthritis.

57. D: Protein-calorie malnutrition, also referred to as PCM, is a deficiency in calories and protein in particular. This disorder is typically the result of an individual eating less; however, it can also occur if the body begins to use up more nutrients than normal. This type of malnutrition is often seen in mild form during most illnesses. More extreme cases of this type of malnutrition can be seen in various disorders. For example, those disorders that cause a reduced nutrient intake include: anorexia, self-induced starvation; dysphagia, inability or difficulty swallowing; gastrointestinal obstructions; and nausea. Disorders that result in the loss of nutrients include diarrhea; glycosuria, glucose in the urine; and hemorrhage. Finally, those that cause the body to use more nutrients than normal include burns, fever, and infection.

58. A: The descending colon is likely to be affected when a patient complains of pain in the left lumbar region. The abdominopelvic cavity is divided in to four regions: Right upper, Left upper, Right lower, and Left lower. Within these regions the abdominopelvic cavity is further divided in to nine sections. By dividing this cavity into sections, healthcare workers are also to communicate clearly about a patient. With regard to the nine sections, these include the right hypochondriac region, epigastric region, left hypochondriac region, Right lumbar region, umbilical region, left lumbar region, Right iliac region, hypogastric region, and the left iliac region.

59. B: The feedback loop is the primary function that maintains homeostasis in the human body. This feedback loop detects when the body is unbalanced and triggers the appropriate mechanisms to bring it back into balance, much like the principles of input and output seen in engineering. Essentially, the nerve endings are the sensors that send messages to the brain, or control center, where the information is processed and acted upon. For example, on a cold day, the skin senses the cold temperature, sends this information to the brain; and the brain tells the muscles (effectors) to shiver, thus bringing the body temperature up. When the body temperature is at the appropriate level, the shivering will stop.

60. C: The plasma membrane's structure is a phospholipid bilayer with proteins. This part of the cell serves as a barrier and protects the cell. On the outer surface of this membrane, protein and carbohydrates have the function of markers to differentiate cells from one another. These components also serve to identify various receptor cells for hormones that will only act on specific cells. The plasma membrane is approximately seven nanometers thick and in addition to protecting the cell, this membrane keeps the cell together with the layers of phospholipid as well as cholesterol that helps stabilize the phospholipids.

61. A: A paper cut will damage the epithelial tissue. Epithelial tissue covers the outside of the body and is a protective barrier. This type of tissue also covers the cavities within the body. The cells of epithelial tissues are packed closely together and cell division is rapid. There are three types of epithelial tissue, cutaneous membrane, serous membrane, and mucous membrane. Cutaneous membranes are the most visible and most abundant in the body, as this type of tissue makes up the skin. Serous membranes are located within closed cavities and have two layers, an epithelial sheet and a layer of simple squamous epithelium. Finally, the mucous membranes are located in cavities that open to the exterior, for example, in the respiratory organs.

62. C: The epiphyseal plate will be the part of the bone that a doctor will look at to determine the adult height of an individual. This structure is made of cartilage and is located between the epiphysis and the diaphysis of the long bone. As the child grows, the epiphyseal plate will begin to harden and when all of the cartilage is harden into bone, growth stops. Once growth stops, what is left is the epiphyseal line marking the point where the epiphysis and the diaphysis have joined. Height can be determined by the thickness of the cartilage, typically by x-raying the wrist.

63. B: The sympathetic system is responsible for responding in emergency situations. This system is a part of the larger autonomic nervous system and is also referred to as the thoracolumbar division. This is often referred to as the fight or flight response. During these situations the sympathetic system will cause a number of other systems or responses to go at the same time. This increased activation of responses allows the body the energy necessary to deal with the stressful situation. Examples of increased responses include sweating, increased heart rate, and secretion of epinephrine, a hormone of the adrenal medulla that reinforces the effects of norepinephrine.

64. C: The muscle pattern that causes the rippled look of a toned stomach is called strap. With this pattern the muscle fibers are aligned and parallel. Other muscle patterns are pinnate, bipennate, multipennate, and triangular, in which fibers are in a diagonal pattern. A fusiform pattern is one in which the fibers are parallel in the belly of the muscle. Spiral and tricipital fibers are twisted and have three muscle bellies, respectively. These patterns are clearly visible and will vary depending on the muscle and its function. For example, the deltoids have a multipennate pattern; the trapezius has a triangular pattern; and the latissimus dorsi has a spiral pattern.

65. D: The possible sprain is contraindicated for massage until a doctor has examined the injury. A sprain can be a stretch, tear, or rip of muscle and can be any one of three grades, or degree of injury. With a mild sprain, Grade 1, the pain is local and tension in the muscle is increased. A moderate or Grade 2 sprain will show indications of reduced or impaired muscle function. With a severe or Grade 3 sprain, there is typically loss of muscle function. It is important to be aware of possible injuries a client may have recently sustained, and while gentle massage may be indicated for such injuries, always have a doctor examine the injury first.

66. B: The most common term in the medical field would be fibromyalgia. It is important for the massage therapist to know and understand medical terminology because it is the key to understanding the body and its pathology. This terminology is the means to speak a common language, which is familiar to all healthcare professionals. Miscommunications in terminology can lead to misunderstandings or more severe consequences to the patient. Understanding medical terminology will also help the therapist when writing treatment notes. When learning medical terminology, consider the parts of the word, for example, Fibro-, meaning fiber or fibrous and my-, meaning muscle. Knowing this we know that the term fibromyalgia is referring to the fibrous muscle tissue. The suffix, -algia means pain. Therefore, when a client states they have fibromyalgia, the therapist will know to be cautious not to cause more pain during the massage.

67. A: Cysts on the kidneys is a symptom rather than a part of the disease's etiology. The definition of etiology is then the incidence or situation in which a disease may occur. In this example, polycystic kidney disease is often hereditary with most cases exhibiting a mutation of the PKD1 gene. Additionally, research suggests that approximately 5% of patients with polycystic kidney disease are in end-stage renal disease. The etiology of a disease will vary depending on the disease, and may include anything from genetics to environmental causes. For example, emphysema, a respiratory disease, may have an etiology of environmental causes.

68. A: Tuberculosis is an airborne illness, meaning the disease is spread through the air, especially when an individual with the disease coughs or sneezes. For contagious diseases, there are a number of ways that the disease can be transmitted: through the air, blood, saliva, or sexual fluids. In order to prevent the healthcare workers from acquiring the disease, they must wear a mask. Blood-borne diseases may be spread through IV drug use, blood transfusions, or cuts. For a massage therapist, the best way to protect themselves from these types of illnesses is to be cautious and aware any cuts on their hands. If cuts or openings are present, then they should either wait until the cut is healed to massage or wear gloves.

69. B: Signs can be observed and measured. Coughing blood, fever, chills, and weight loss, all can be seen by outside observers and measures. On the other hand, chest pain would be referred to as a symptom, which is something that is subjective and only felt by the patient. Diseases contain both signs and symptoms and these words are often used interchangeably. As a massage therapist, you will never diagnose an individual, however if someone complains to you about various symptoms or you see signs that are questionable, you can also suggest they see their primary care physician.

70. A: Massage releases serotonin as well as dopamine. The release of serotonin regulates moods and allows the appropriate emotions to be displayed during any specific situation. Serotonin also effects in the individual in terms of calming. In an individual with depression, their serotonin is low. When serotonin is released, it may level out the depressed mood. Other psychological issues such as obsessive-compulsive disorders, chronic pain disorders, and eating disorders are also indicated by lower levels of serotonin, and may therefore benefit from massage. It is always important for a massage therapist to be aware of psychological problems and medication their clients are on, as some have adverse reactions to a calming massage.

71. C: The most appropriate massage technique for individuals with autism would be a firm, purposeful touch. These individuals, while some would think counter-intuitively, do like and want to be touched. However, for individuals with autism, their development disability is one in which social interactions are hindered and their days consist of a series of deliberate actions and behaviors. Therefore, massage should also be as such in order to make the client feel comfortable. Most importantly, a massage therapist must always respect the client and remain in constant communication during the massage, to ensure they are having a comfortable and beneficial experience.

72. A: Massage in general will influence the automatic nervous system and in a relaxation massage, this can be very calming, thus reducing the amount of anxiety felt by the client. Massage therapists must always remember to begin with a client based on where they are personally. For example, if a client comes into a massage with heightened anxiety, they may be resistant to gentle slow strokes at first. Therefore, the therapist should communicate with and respect the client in order to create a massage that is beneficial for them and helps ease their anxiety.

73. A: Individuals with osteoporosis have a serious bone disease. This disease results in a loss of bone density, specifically the loss of calcium, and is most typical in postmenopausal women. While its direct cause is unknown, osteoporosis has been linked to a decrease in the female hormone estrogen. Literally translated, osteoporosis means a porous bone. In some individuals, the condition will have progressed to a point where bone fractures can occur with no or little impact. Therefore, it is important for a therapist to be aware of any condition and adjust their massage accordingly.

74. B: The informed consent is the form required that gives the therapist permission to work on an individual. This form must be signed by a consenting adult or, in the case of body work for a minor, a legal guardian. It is important that the informed consent provides information about the nature of massage as well as information indicating that the individual has the right to refuse treatment at any point during the massage. By providing clients with this information, they have the opportunity to make an educated, informed decision on whether they want to receive treatment.

75. C: Transference occurs during a client-therapist relationship when the client transfers personal feelings onto the therapist. In this case the client may be seeing you as so much like their deceased spouse that they begin feeling for you what they felt of their spouse. As a massage therapist, this issue should be dealt with professionally and with sensitivity. If the client is unable to deal with these feelings in a healthy way, it would be most responsible for the therapist to refer the client to another massage therapist and/or grief counseling so they could learn to deal with the death of their spouse.

76. D: Countertransference occurs when a therapist places personal feelings on to their client. In this case as a therapist also recently dealing with the death of a loved one, you may find that your client reminds you of the deceased. It could also be that because of the similarities in your situations you may feel a superficial connection and attribute that connection to something deep. In this case, the best solution may be to be honest with your client and refer them to a different therapist.

77. B: Massaging your client's face would be crossing their personal boundaries. Personal boundaries will be different for everyone, and it is important to learn what these boundaries are for each client before beginning a massage. These are boundaries that we all set for ourselves on how close someone can get before we are no longer comfortable. In this situation, because your client stated prior to the massage that they did not like having their face massaged, then this clearly is a personal boundary. If a massage therapist ignores these things, then the massage will become an unpleasant experience for the client. Additionally, not all clients will say out loud what their boundaries are. By paying attention and watching for signs of discomfort, a therapist can ask questions and modify the massage to make sure the client is comfortable.

78. C: Listening and offering your own assessment of your client's situation is beyond a massage therapist's scope of practices and therefore would be considered crossing a legal and ethical boundary. It is important for a massage therapist to be empathic and show concern and sensitivity, especially for clients in vulnerable positions. However, a therapist can cause unwarranted damage if they offer services that they are unqualified to provide. In situations where a therapist crosses a legal boundary, they are at risk for not only harming their clients, but also harming their practice and may face legal actions.

79. A: Medical terminology is a set of terms, typically Latin or Greek that provides all healthcare professionals a common language. While not all massage therapists will work directly with a chiropractor or other medical professional, it will still be important for all to understand and know how to properly use medical terminology. There may be times throughout your career that you encounter a client with various health needs. In some cases, a physician, or other healthcare professional consultation will be necessary in order for you to provide the best and safest care to your client.

80. C: An independent contractor essentially is their own boss. While, as an independent contractor you may rent a room from a spa, you are still responsible for paying all of your own taxes; however, the rent you pay for the room rental could be deducted as a business expense. Independent contractors must keep careful records of all of their profits and losses, as all will be included on schedule C of their tax forms. In addition to keeping records, independent contractors are required to pay quarterly taxes, which is typically one quarter of the tax you expect to owe by the end of the year.

81. B: While not required in many European countries, draping is required by law for massage in the United States. This is a way the massage therapist can maintain their client's privacy and ensure the client is comfortable and warm throughout the massage. There are various techniques for draping; however, the main focus is to uncover only the body part you are working on. As noted, draping is also used to keep the client warm. Since as the client relaxes their body temperature may decrease, it is very easy to become cold during a massage. With this additional point in mind, therapists should also have extra blankets on hand.

82. A: Endangerment sites are locations on the body where the nerves are superficial. Pressure on these areas may cause the client extreme discomfort or potential damage to the underlying vessels and nerves. In addition to the armpit, the following are also considered endangerment sites: the eyes, inferior to the ear, the posterior cervical area, lymph nodes, the medial brachium, musculocutaneous nerve, median nerve, ulnar nerve, basilic vein, cubital areas of the median nerve, and radial and ulnar arteries and under the knees. Light strokes over these areas may be allowable; however, a massage therapist must always be careful and watch for signs of discomfort.

83. C: When discussing various conditions in terms of severity, healthcare workers will typically refer to the condition as acute or chronic. In this case, the back pain is chronic because it is existed for about a year. Had the client stated that his back problems began last week, the condition would be considered acute. Acute conditions will typically be short in duration; however, if a condition continues, it can become a chronic problem. As a massage therapist, it is important to understand if a client's conditions are acute or chronic so you know how to treat and track the problem.

84. C: If a client comes for a massage and is ill, the best thing of their therapist to do would be to refer them to a physician. Referrals are necessary in some cases because the therapist is not qualified to diagnosis or treat diseases. Referrals can also be used to enhance the client's treatment and healing. For example, you may refer a client to a chiropractor and suggest they have their back adjusted immediately following a massage. This would enhance the client's healing process. Because referrals are common in this field, it is important for therapists to be familiar with the various healthcare professionals in their area.

85. A: Confidentiality is the client's right to privacy. According to the Health Insurance Portability and Accountability Act of 1996, all healthcare professionals are required to maintain their client's confidentiality, which includes all massage therapists. When a new client comes in for a massage, it is the therapist's responsibility to inform the client about confidentiality and their rights to privacy. While therapists must maintain confidentiality, there may be situations were discussing a case is allowable; for example, when consulting with other healthcare professionals, if they are discussing clients with a supervisor for training or evaluation purposes, or if required by law.

86. B: S.O.A.P refers to Subjective Objective Assessment and Plan. With this form of note taking, the therapist will provide a range of information beginning with subjective information. This will consist completely of information that the client provides to the therapist. The subjective information will be what the therapist finds after working on the client. This could include information such as range of motion or observed signs of disorder. The assessment section of the documentation will include the outcomes of the session, for medical doctors, this section would include a diagnosis. Finally, the plan section of these notes will discuss the treatment plan.

87. C: Lymphatic massage would be contraindicated by a malignant neoplasm because this is a tumor or cancer that can be spread. Such tumors are abnormal growths, often caused by genetic conditions and are registered by the rest of the body as parasites. In many cases malignant neoplasms are spread through the lymphatic system and if massage if performed, the therapists may spread this disease to other parts of the body. The other type of tumor is a benign tumor, which is not spreadable. These tumors typically grow slower then malignant tumors and only become life-threatening if they grow to a size that hinders the functioning of surrounding organs.

88. A: Sprains are injuries to ligaments and are classified in three grades. In this case, the sprain would be classified as a Grade 1 sprain, which is mild and includes 0%-20% fiber tear. With this grade, the individual will continue to have normal range of motion by the area may be tender and slightly swollen. A Grade 2 sprain refers to a 20%-75% fiber tear, moderate resistance, swelling, muscle splinting, and a reduced range of motion. The final type of sprain is a Grade 3 sprain and refers to a 75%-100% fiber tear. This is a severe sprain that is painful and little to no motion.

89. C: Strains are injuries to muscles and tendons and are classified in three degrees. A first-degree strain results in 0%-10% fiber tear, mild pain and tenderness, and swelling. With a first-degree strain, the individual usually still has all normal functioning. A second-degree strain results in a 10%-50% fiber tear, pain, swelling, muscle splinting, and a reduced functioning. Finally, a third-degree strain results in a 50%-100% fiber tear, severe pain, swelling, and little to no muscle functioning. Regardless of the degree of the strain, massage is contraindicated for at least the first 24 hours after the injury and it may be beneficial for the therapist to refer the client for further evaluation and treatment prior to massaging the strained area.

90. B: A complete fracture is one in which the bone becomes completely separated. In addition to this type of fracture, other types of fractures include incomplete, closed, open, comminuted, compression, stress, greenstick, nonunion, malunion, delayed union, and spiral fractures. Of the more common fractures, the incomplete fracture results in a crack that does not go all the way through the bone. A closed fracture affects the bone but not the skin, while an open fracture affects both the bone and skin. A comminuted fracture results in the bone being cracked or splintered in more than one piece and a compression fracture is when the bone is pushed together, resulting in a fracture.

91. D: Cervicogenic headaches are related to various trigger points and would benefit from this type of massage. Symptoms of cervicogenic headaches may include altered neck posture and a limited range of motion. Other headache types include migraine, cluster, tension, and chronic daily. Migraine headaches are severe headaches with symptoms such as nausea and vomiting, extreme sensitivity to light, and eye pain. Cluster headaches are similar to migraine except these occur in clusters. Tension headaches are caused by muscle tension and may be relieved by massage; these headaches are not as severe as migraines. Chronic daily headaches can be caused from a number of things and specific treatment will depend on the cause of these headaches.

92. B: Hypovolemic shock is the result of a large amount of blood causing a decrease in blood pressure. While a hemorrhage is the most common cause of hypovolemic shock, the loss of interstitial fluid may also cause this type of shock. Cardiogenic shock may result from a variety of types of heart failure. Neurogenic shock results from the dilation of blood vessels, creating an unstable autonomic stimulation of smooth muscles. Anaphylactic shock is caused by an allergic reaction. A fifth type of shock includes a septic shock that is the result of septicemia, or the release of infectious toxins in the body.

93. D: Bronchitis is a lower respiratory tract infection because it occurs in the bronchi. With bronchitis, there is swelling of the bronchi due to infection and often the trachea is also infected. In these cases the disease is referred to as tracheobronchitis. This disease causes deep cough, typically with mucus and pus. Other lower respiratory tract infections include pneumonia, which is an infection in the lungs. Tuberculosis is a contagious disease that affects the lungs and surrounding tissues. Emphysema is caused from chronic bronchitis causing the alveoli to enlarge and rupture. Finally, asthma is the result of muscle spasms in the smooth muscles of the bronchial passages.

94. B: Hypernatremia is caused by sodium imbalance; specifically too much sodium. This is typically defined as above 145 mEq/L. Hypernatremia could be cause by a high salt diet and may result in dehydration or diarrhea. On the other hand, hyponatremia would be too little sodium; typically below 136 mEq/L. Sodium imbalances affect the nervous system and include symptoms such as confusion, headaches, seizures, coma, and death. Potassium imbalances include levels less than 3.8 mEq/L and above 5.1 mEq/L. Small imbalances of potassium can result in serious illnesses. Calcium imbalances include any level less than 8.4 mg/dL or more than 10.5 mg/dL. Symptoms of calcium imbalances include muscle weakness, reduced reflexes, pancreatitis, and rickets.

95. B: The purpose of the massage therapist and the massage itself is to increase cell metabolism, decrease pain, and increase range of motion. It is not to heal. All healthcare professionals must work within the scope of their practice. For a massage therapist, diagnosing and treating disease is out of their scope of practice. However, many massage techniques will help with the healing process and it is beneficial if the therapist is in communication with the client's physician if they are being treated for other illnesses or conditions. This communication will provide the client with the best possible care.

96. A: Breaking up adhesions is considered a mechanical effect of massage. Mechanical effects are the result of applying direct pressure to the body. Other ways to create mechanical effects include assisted stretching techniques. Physiological effects are those that result in physical and chemical changes in the body. For example, a massage may help flush toxins and other waste products, which would increase blood flow and cellular metabolism. Psychological effects create an emotional change in the body. With massage, stimulation of the nervous system can reduce stress and increase relaxation and well being.

97. B: The lymphatic system relies on voluntary muscle movement in order to be moved throughout the body. This movement is important, as it is the lymph that is responsible for carrying waste and toxins from cell breakdown and metabolism out of the body. Massage is beneficial with this process, as it can assist with this movement. Just as massage increases blood circulation, it also increases lymphatic circulation. In addition, the flow of lymph out of the blood stream also increases because massage tends to open closed blood capillaries through the release of histamines and acetylcholine.

98. C: A muscle spasm or cramps can occur with overstimulation of the nervous system. In order to release a muscle spasm or cramp, it is suggested that the therapist perform compressions on the tendon of the muscle. This technique activates proprioceptors, which in turn release the spasm or cramp. Other techniques include slow stretching, stimulation of the Golgi tendons, and reciprocal inhibition treatments. Golgi tendons monitor the length of the muscles and react accordingly in order to bring a muscle back to normal. If the Golgi tendon senses that the muscle is overextended, it will contract; on the other hand, if the Golgi tendon senses that the muscle is too contracted, it will relax. In addition, Golgi tendons have inhibitory effects on muscles in order to maintain the normal position of the muscle.

99. C: Effleurage or gliding is typically the first stroke of a massage. This stroke helps to warm the muscles and help relax the client. With this massage stroke, the therapist's hands are firm but relaxed, and glide easily over the muscles. This stroke can also be used with the therapist's forearms, thumbs, or fists. Therapists should keep in mind that the effleurage stroke should be consistent in speed and pressure. Other uses for this massage stroke include to apply oil, assess your client's muscles, establish your client's pressure tolerance, stimulate muscles, stretch muscles, and to increase lymphatic flow.

100. A: Petrissage or kneading focuses on the deeper tissue and may involve lifting, rolling, and compressing the deep muscles. This stroke type is used sparingly as it can be exhausting for the therapist, however, proper body mechanics can assist in endurance. Petrissage strokes also include skin rolling, fulling, and ischemic compression. Petrissage is beneficial to the client in a number of ways including, increasing the removal of metabolic waste and other toxins, release adhesions in muscle bellies, increasing the flow of fluid in deep tissue, and stretching muscle tissue and fascia.

101. A: Range of motion is the natural movement that a joint can go through. Depending on the joint, its range of motion will vary. For example, The cervical joint has a range of motion from 0-80 degrees, shoulder from 0-180 degrees, elbow 0-140 degrees, radioulnar from 0-80 degrees, wrist from 0- 60, thoracic from 0-50 degrees, lumbar from 0-60 degrees, hip from 0-100 degrees, knee from 0-150 degrees, ankle from 0-40 degrees, subtalar from 0-30 degrees, and the metatarsophalangeal from 0-50 degrees. Note that the normal range of motion will also vary for each joint depending on the type of movement (e.g., flexion, extension, etc.). When a joint has abnormal restrictions its range of motion is reduced.

102. A: Massage is indicated for the treatment of asthma, as massage may be helpful in reducing stress and loosening intercostals, thus increasing breathing. Other conditions are contraindicated for massage and could result in further injury or problems. Edema, which is swelling, can be caused by a number of things; the massage therapist should ask questions in order to figure the cause, In the cases of edema due to heart decompensations, infection, kidney ailments, or obstructions, massage is contraindicated. Bursitis is inflammation of the bursae, and massage could increase the inflammatory response. Abdominal aneurysm is contraindicated on the abdomen. The therapist can massage other parts of the body not affected.

103. B: A systemic effect of hydrotherapy will affect the entire body. For example, vasodilation causes a drop in blood pressure throughout the entire body. A therapist may create a systemic effect by applying heat for 20-30 minutes. This heat application will continue to produce effects for up to an hour after the treatment. Local effects are restricted to specific areas of the body. Reflex affects the skin and other body parts through the nervous system. The various types of effects apply to both hot and cold applications. The results will depend on the type of treatment.

104. C: The study of movement is called Kinesiology. This field is often combined with biomechanics which looks at movement in terms of mechanics. Within this field, muscles are classified or termed according to their function. Prime movers are the muscles that initiate and maintain movement. Synergists assist the prime movers. Antagonists oppose the prime movers. The combination of a prime mover and an antagonist is referred to as a fixator. There are also neutralizers that inhibit unwarranted movement while the prime mover is in action. In addition to their functional classifications, there are different characteristics of muscles, including fast, slow, and intermediate twitch muscle fibers.

105. D: Specialized testing may include passive or active range of motion (ROM), strength testing, or orthopedic testing. The purpose of specialized tests is to determine the functionality of various areas of the body. Other parts of this type of assessment include taking a history including the client's family medical history, and personal medical history. Observations are also useful and should include mood, gait, and standing and sitting postures. A final component of this assessment includes palpation, which begins with the superficial tissue and gradually moves to the deeper tissues. With palpation, the therapist will feel for symmetry, temperature, muscle tone, and texture.

106. C: Microvilli are found only in the small intestine and are organelles within the cytoplasmic membrane. The function of the microvilli is to increase the surface area of the small intestines and assist in absorption. These microvilli are a part of an extensive network of organelles that absorb fats from chime. Included in this process are lacteal, which are lymphatic vessels; plicae, circular folds; and villi, finger-like projections; all serving to increase the surface area of the small intestine and facilitate absorption. As materials enter into the small intestine, they travel through the duodenum, where most of the absorption occurs to the jejunum, and finally the ileum.

107. C: The permease system also called a cell or ion pump moves molecules against the concentration gradient. Because this movement is against the gradient, energy or ATP is required, thus it is an active transport system. Other active transport systems include pinocytosis, in which a cell will engulf liquid droplets and process them; and phagocytosis, or cell eating, in which a cell will engulf a solid molecule and process it. With phagocytosis, a cell will typically engulf bacteria or other cellular waste. Since ATP is required for these processes, the cells exert work and require chemical processes in order to create the energy required.

108. B: Amy will have to pay out-of-pocket expenses for the flood damage because she did not purchase Business & Personal Property Loss insurance. This type of insurance covers a business owner for a number of events including fires, water damage, or theft. Had Amy purchased this type of insurance, the insurance would have covered the loss of any business or personal equipment. While some events seem unlikely, it is important to understand the risks involved in owning a business as well as the precautions one can take to protect all business and personal assets.

109. B: Amy is covered in this case because she has Property Damage and Bodily Injury Liability. With this type of insurance, incidents that occur at her office including falls or slips as well as injury due to equipment failure are covered. This type of insurance is required in many states and may be specifically be required by a landlord if a therapist rents office space for their practice. In addition to covering a client in the case of an accident, this insurance protects the therapist from unwarranted bills or legal actions.

110. C: Amy did not develop a business plan. This is an essential document for any business, as it includes important information about the business, and its mission and goals. A typical business plan will include the following information: cover page, table of contents, owner's statement, executive summary, purpose and goals, a detailed description of the business, a marketing plan, risk assessment and financial analysis, operations and organizational policies, strategies for success, and other supporting information that the owner feels is necessary. While others may not read this document, it is important to have and keep updated in order to ensure you are on track with your business goals and you are able to refine these goals as the business grows.

111. B: By creating a logo and marketing materials, Amy is developing her professional image. Your professional image is the outward image presented to the public and your clients. It is important for therapists to represent themselves in a professional manner. Other ways a massage therapist can develop their professional image include keeping a clean massage room and waiting room, proper dress attire, and efficient and professional communication skills. A therapist's professional image will also expand to the therapeutic session itself, those who keep accurate notes, listen and are empathic toward their clients and respect their clients privacy show a positive professional image.

112. C: The occupational therapist would be the best referral in this case. The role of an occupational therapist is to work with clients to increase independence, thus increasing their quality of life. This type of therapist focuses on activities typically performed at work, in the home, or related to self care. It is an Occupational Therapist's job to enhance the development of their clients functioning. While you may continue to work with the client, the referral and continued communication with the other therapist would be essential in providing the client the best care possible.

113. A: Airway, Breathing, Circulation are the ABCs of First Aid. This is considered the primary survey and should be conducted immediately after finding a victim. If the individual is in any immediate danger, First Aid protocol states that you address any problem and then move on a secondary survey or assessment. The secondary survey will be more thorough and will include a full body survey to search for any injuries. It is important that both the primary and the secondary surveys are completed and are efficient as these precautions could be life-saving as the victim waits for emergency medical help.

114. B: An asymmetric standing position is the most efficient position for a massage therapist. For this position, the therapist will stand with one foot in front of the other. This will allow the therapist to leverage their own body weight into the massage. Additionally, as body weight is shifted from one foot to the other, the therapist can conserve energy. This position also protects the ankle and foot and allows for the knees to be bent throughout the massage. It is also beneficial to sit when possible while performing massage in order to conserve energy.

115. B: Passive joint movements also referred to as arthrokinematic movement occur as a result of another movement. This type of passive movement could also be considered the "play" a joint has or its ability to move freely within the joint capsule. Typically resulting after active movements, this accessory movement may slide, roll, or spin within a joint. On the other hand, active joint movements, or osteokinematic movements are voluntary and require effort to perform. For example flexing the arm is considered an osteokinematic movement. In massage, the therapist may perform various movements through stretching.

116. C: The anatomic barrier is the point at which injury would occur to a joint. Each joint's anatomic barrier will vary and is expressed as degrees for range of motion. However, because it is at this barrier that injury will occur, other barriers exist to avoid reaching the anatomic barrier. The physiologic barrier is determined by sensory functions of the nervous system. The physiologic barrier allows for full range of motion and full functionality of the joint. In addition to this barrier, there is the pathologic barrier that hinders normal range of motion. This may be expressed as stiffness or pain in the joint.

117. B: All massage therapists should have a basic understanding of the functions and dysfunctions of the human body. However, for those therapists who are interested in working with physicians or within other medical settings, it will be even more important to understand these elements of the human body. It will be in these settings that the massage therapist will encounter a variety of illnesses and dysfunctions. As such, they must understand the indications, contraindications, and precautions that must be taken for each of their clients. These therapists may choose additional training in medical massage to ensure that they are knowledgeable to practice in this specialized field.

118. C: The effects of hydrotherapy are seen mostly within the autonomic nervous system. Depending upon the temperature of the water being used for the therapy, different aspects of this system will be stimulated. For example, to stimulate the sympathetic system, the therapist will use cold water, while they will use warm water to stimulate the parasympathetic responses. Additionally, by applying heat or cold for varying periods of time, the therapist can affect the dilatation of the circulatory system. More specifically, cold application for a short period of time will stimulate the nervous system and cause vasoconstriction.

119. C: Lymphatic drainage focuses on this system and helps move various toxins out of the body. While this is done naturally, manually manipulating the lymphatic system may cause a toxin overload and affect the client, causing them to feel fatigued. There are various modifications of lymphatic drainage including techniques developed my Emil Vodder, Eyal Lederman, and Bruno Chickly. However, regardless of the style used, this is a specialized massage technique that requires additional training. Lymph moves through the body through lymph vessels that are not controlled by the heart pump. Therefore the lymph vessels must contract in order to move the lymph through. Lymphatic drainage is one way to assist this system and drain toxins from the body.

120. B: Low blood pressure is contraindicated for lymphatic drainage because this type of body work lowers blood pressure. By performing for lymphatic drainage on a client who already has low blood pressure, dizziness and fainting may occur upon standing after the bodywork. Other contraindications include illnesses; both viral and bacterial infections. These are contraindicated because the lymphatic drainage may spread the illness to other parts of the body, thus enhancing the illness. In clients with fever, lymphatic drainage lowers body temperature. Finally, this type of body work affects the client's circulation and therefore those clients with weak hearts or other heart conditions may be contraindicated for lymphatic drainage.

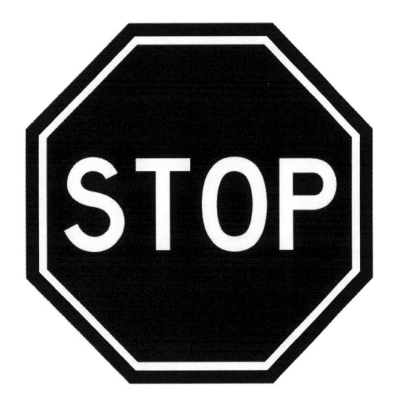

FREE Test Taking Tips DVD Offer

To help us better serve you, we have developed a Test Taking Tips DVD that we would like to give you for <u>FREE</u>. **This DVD covers world-class test taking tips that you can use to be even more successful when you are taking your test.**

All that we ask is that you email us your feedback about your study guide. Please let us know what you thought about it – whether that is good, bad or indifferent.

To get your **FREE Test Taking Tips DVD**, email <u>freedvd@studyguideteam.com</u> with "FREE DVD" in the subject line and the following information in the body of the email:

    a. The title of your study guide.

    b. Your product rating on a scale of 1-5, with 5 being the highest rating.

    c. Your feedback about the study guide. What did you think of it?

    d. Your full name and shipping address to send your free DVD.

If you have any questions or concerns, please don't hesitate to contact us at <u>freedvd@studyguideteam.com</u>.

Thanks again!

39472319R00062

Made in the USA
San Bernardino, CA
26 September 2016